The Man in the Arena:
Surviving Multiple Myeloma Since 1992

To Brian –
  Don't be a d--k to your
nurses. Good luck with
everything!

   Best wishes –
     Elaim..... um....
I mean.......Author Guy.

Published by BookLocker.com, Inc., St. Petersburg, Florida.

Printed on acid-free paper.

BookLocker.com, Inc.
2021

First Edition

Author contact Information: The author can be reached at jim.bond48@gmail.com

Dedication

This book is dedicated to the memory of our departed parents, Delores J. and James E. Bond, and our departed sister, Janell. They are my heroes.

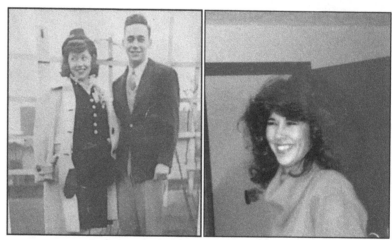

Delores and the original James Bond
Our wonderful sister, Janell

DISCLAIMER

This book details the author's memory of personal experiences with and opinions about surviving multiple myeloma since 1992. The author is not a healthcare provider.

The author and publisher are providing this book and its contents on an "as is" basis and make no representations or warranties of any kind with respect to this book or its contents. The author and publisher disclaim all such representations and warranties, including for example warranties of merchantability and healthcare for a particular purpose. In addition, the author and publisher do not represent or warrant that the information accessible via this book is accurate, complete or current.

The statements made about products and services have not been evaluated by the U.S. Food and Drug Administration. They are not intended to diagnose, treat, cure, or prevent any condition or disease. Please consult with your own physician or healthcare specialist regarding the suggestions and recommendations made in this book.

Except as specifically stated in this book, neither the author or publisher, nor any authors, contributors, or other representatives will be liable for damages arising out of or in connection with the use of this book. This is a comprehensive limitation of liability that applies to all damages of any kind, including (without limitation) compensatory; direct, indirect or consequential damages; loss of data, income or profit; loss of or damage to property and claims of third parties.

You understand that this book is not intended as a substitute for consultation with a licensed healthcare practitioner, such as your physician. Before you begin any healthcare program, or change your lifestyle in any way, you will consult your physician or other licensed healthcare practitioner to ensure that you are in good health and that the examples contained in this book will not harm you.

This book provides content related to topics physical and/or mental health issues. As such, use of this book implies your acceptance of this disclaimer.

Table of Contents

Introduction

This true story is written by a long-term survivor of a deadly, incurable blood cancer called multiple myeloma (also referred to as myeloma). In the US, there are an estimated 100,000 to 200,000+ myeloma patients alive at any time. When the author was diagnosed, the average survival was about 3 years, and it currently is about 7 years, thanks to several new ground-breaking myeloma drugs. The author was in initial clinical trials that helped two of the most widely used new myeloma drugs gain FDA approval, and are used worldwide.

There are other long-term myeloma survivors, but not enough. The author believes there will be more long-term survivors due to continued research, new drugs, and treatments.

Each case is unique, and this one case does not imply otherwise. How each patient chooses to treat myeloma is also unique to the patient, their family, and their medical team.

Who We Are

I am the real James Bond, but I am not a movie actor. My proof is that I've been married to my best friend and the most beautiful 'Bond Girl', Kathleen, for over 50 years.

Kathleen and I met at Ohio University where I was in the Business College and she was in the Communications College. I studied hard to earn the top ranking in my business class.

I admired Kathy Mercer (now Kathleen Bond) and finally met her in our OU cafeteria. The topic of baseball came up and I asked Kathy if she had ever heard of Hall of Fame pitcher Satchel Paige and his famous hesitation pitch. She surprised me that she was aware of Satchel and that she could throw his hesitation pitch. We met behind my dorm, and I tossed Kathleen a hardball and a glove. Some of my dorm-mates were watching from the windows. She amazed me by throwing a good hesitation pitch. More than five decades later she continues to do amazing things.

The Vietnam war was raging when I graduated, but I received a draft deferment for an old sports injury. Suddenly, our future opened; going to war was no longer a barrier. We decided to get married, even though we had not really planned that far into the future. Kathleen hoped to complete her last college year in Boston, where I accepted a job offer from Ernst & Ernst, now EY.

Kathleen's college plans took a slight detour when our first son Jim, arrived a year after our wedding. A few years after Jim, our second son Bob was born. My career was going well and after 5 years in our Boston office, I was selected for transfer to our headquarters in Cleveland, Ohio. It was a three-year assignment, working with EY's leaders. With the assurance I could resume my Boston job after the three years, we accepted the transfer and moved to a Cleveland suburb. Both of our parents and some siblings were now near us in the Akron area which was an added benefit.

While my career was demanding, my family was my top priority. I was determined to balance my job with our young family's needs. For many years, I planned my calendar by first scheduling a family vacation rental in remote Cape Hatteras for late summer. With a deposit already paid, it was easier for EY partners to accept that I was unavailable during my vacation to spend time with my wife and our sons. It may have slowed down my promotion progress a bit, but I was confident in my career and contributions to the firm. I realized being with Kathleen and our young sons while they were growing up happened only once. Watching Jim and Bob play different sports and just hanging out meant a lot to me, and it still does to this day.

Kathleen volunteered at the boy's grade school, the American Cancer Society (ACS), and other non-profit organizations. While I briefly coached at the grade school, Kathleen coached more frequently. She helped to break the gender barrier as one of the first women coaches of the girl's junior high basketball team despite the fact that we didn't have daughters or that she knew little about coaching basketball.

When our sons became more independent, Kathleen enrolled in nearby John Carroll University. She jokingly called herself the "old lady" among her younger classmates. One professor, labeled her "the wily housewife" for her consistently top test scores. The last year she missed at Ohio University due to our wedding and relocation turned into several years at JCU. Kathleen ran our household while taking a class or two at a time. I am very proud that Kathleen graduated summa cum laude. Her commencement was within a week of Jim's high school graduation, which was a great celebration for our family. Not only did she juggle the household, college classes, and our son's activities, her hard work and leadership skills were becoming recognized in charitable circles.

I kept myself in physical shape by playing with Bob and Jim and jogging before work or during my lunch hour. I also did all our yard work and several home remodeling and maintenance projects, some of which I had help from my Dad. I learned remodeling skills growing up and working in the summer for my Grandfather or Dad, who was our family's first James Bond. They both were self-employed plastering contractors, but Dad branched out to other remodeling projects. When I was a teenager, my mother Delores told me I would not follow my Dad's occupation. Being self-employed meant uncertainty of when the next job was coming. She said, "You will go to college and get a good office job". This was her strong advice and I am thankful for her direction to this day.

My mother was a trailblazer. When my three sisters and I were old enough to be home alone, Mom began working as a bank teller. During her career, she was selected as the Akron, Ohio area's first drive-in window teller. My parents and grandparents took time to teach me valuable life lessons, including to work hard and face challenges head on.

When Mom was only 57, she passed away from ovarian and breast cancer that spread to her liver. It was awful to watch my mother lie in her hospital bed and to see my father and sisters grieve. Earlier, Kathleen and I turned down EY's option to transfer back to Boston after my three-year assignment in the Cleveland National office. Being so close to our parents and siblings provided more time to be together which was important to us. This was especially true for my mother who loved being with our sons. We created lasting family memories living so close to each other.

Unfortunately, more bad news came to our family. Just a few short months after the birth of her first child, my sister Janell passed away from cancer in 1992. Melanoma, a type of skin cancer, had quickly spread to several organs. Her husband Charlie was devastated, and our entire family was in shock. Janell was told her melanoma spot which had been removed ten years earlier would not come back. However, being pregnant may have triggered the return of her cancer. Janell said in one of her last days, if that were the case, she would do it again. She said it was worth it for her to have a child with her husband, Charlie. Janell and I were close throughout her life and losing her was heart breaking.

To our family, cancer meant death.

Our World Changed

A few months after Janell passed, I had my E&Y required physical exam at one of our 2 major hospitals in Cleveland. Kathleen was glad I was complying, since she thought I was looking pale, 'even for an accountant', as she quipped. I had a slight ache in my lower back, but thought we may just need a new mattress. When the exam was complete, the diligent doctor said they saw nothing in my exam to worry about, but he wanted to follow-up on one test result. I thought he was being very fussy, but that was not the case.

My urine showed excess protein, but the doctor said sometimes it happens with joggers like me. He ordered more tests, including x-rays of my kidneys which looked good. However, the doctor asked me if I was born with rounded lower spine vertebrae which the x-ray showed, instead of normal squared-off ones. I said I had never been told that was the case, but my lower back and ribs did ache slightly. He then asked me to see a hematologist/oncologist (hem/onc). When Kathleen heard my news, she was not as surprised as I had been. She had suspected I may have a serious problem, but prayed it was stress from our recent loss of Janell.

We both attended the hem/onc appointment. Alan Lichtin was pleasant and fairly young. He wanted me to get a bone marrow biopsy to determine what was causing my mis-shaped vertebrae and excess urine protein. Bone marrow biopsies involved lying on my stomach, having a large needle pushed into my hip bone, and extracting a marrow sample for analysis. Some were more painful than others.

The doctor reviewed the biopsy results, met with us, and explained, "Unfortunately, you have a cancer called Multiple Myeloma (myeloma)."

I had never heard of myeloma, but it was what Kathleen feared from her medical library research (1992 was pre-internet). Alan further explained that my case was at the most advanced stage. My skull had advanced lytic lesions and I had broken ribs and other bone damage, including my vertebrae. Kathleen was wiping tears from her eyes, and I was stunned. Our world was turned upside down. The bomb 'hit me,' but she was collateral damage, as she accurately said.

I asked the hem/onc if myeloma had a cure and I was told there was no cure. I asked, "How long do you believe I will live, doctor?" Alan did not want to answer, but I persisted until he said, "If you do nothing, you will live a few months, if you do all you can, maybe 3 years, *if all goes well.*"

If all goes well, 3 years! His words hung in the air.

Although we were reeling, I managed to ask, "If you were in my shoes, what would you do?"

He paused, then said, "I would consider retiring and doing my bucket list while I still could."

I managed one last question, "If you were me, whom would you have treat your case, and don't limit your choices to Cleveland?" This question seemed to surprise Alan as he sat back in his chair and finally said, "At nearby Case Western Reserve Medical School (Case), my excellent hematology professor, Bob Kellermeyer (Bob K) is whom I would see. He is a hem/onc who practices across the street at the other major cancer center, University Hospitals (UH) of Cleveland. Bob sees more myeloma cases than I do."

UH is a teaching hospital, affiliated with the Case Medical School. From her ACS volunteer work, Kathleen knew UH was one of only 2 National Cancer Center (NCI) designated comprehensive cancers in Ohio. The other is in Columbus.

I expected Alan to say he was the right doctor for me, and really respected that he was placing my health above his practice and his hospital. He helped me get an appointment with Bob K the next day. Alan's compassion impacted my EY career. Was I responding to client requests with similar compassion for them? From that day, I tried to better address problems from my client's perspective.

Alan's 1992 recommendation was key to my survival. About 15 years later, after we shared our survival story at his hospital's support group, I spotted Alan and asked him if he recalls his response to have Bob K, rather than himself, treat me. He said "no", but he lowered his voice and added, "Please don't let my leader over there hear that I did this."

His leader is our friend and has moved on to lead another out of town cancer center. I am still in contact with Alan.

Our Best Shot

The days after hearing my dire diagnosis were very hard. We seriously considered retiring and completing our 'bucket list', but truth be told, we really didn't't have a list. We had just become empty nesters since Bob joined Jim in college at Miami University in Oxford, Ohio, a few hundred miles from our home. We considered the painful endings of different cancers that took Mom and Janell. Maybe, we wondered, enjoying what may be a short time was better than working.

But I thought about all the great family memories over my life, and I desperately wanted to be part of future memories. Jim, Bob, and I spent hours playing catch, golf, and even basketball in the driveway. We enjoyed watching their sports teams play and had great family gatherings with Kathleen's family and mine. At my sister Denyse's and brother-in-law Charlie's home, we played spirited volleyball and softball games, and even went on a hayride with Charlie pulling the wagon with his tractor. Playing weekly golf after work with my Dad and my sister Becki's husband, Dan Kramer, was priceless.

We had a ball on Cape Hatteras vacations with Kathleen's extended family, and later with my Mom and Dad. There were no telephones, TVs, or other distractions in our remote rented beach house where we fished and played in the surf daily. These and many, many more good times were worth fighting for more. I refused to give up.

I also thought back to overcoming a terrible accident I had as an aspiring high school baseball player. I attended Cuyahoga Falls high school, a large school with about a thousand kids in each grade. I tried out for the varsity baseball team my sophomore year and made the team as our starting third baseman. That year, we won our district and were playing a Cleveland team for a trip to the state finals. I recall making a rookie mental error that cost us the early lead. I somewhat redeemed myself with a hit at my next at bat, but we lost the game. It's not the hit, but the mental mistake, that still sticks with me.

In northeast Ohio, high school baseball is played in our normally cold, wet spring. Early in my junior year, I slipped running the bases on a muddy infield, injuring my hand. I played despite the injury, but had only a mediocre season. We did not return to the state regional playoffs.

With my hand healed, I played much better on our summer team, which won the right to represent Akron in a high-profile Cincinnati tournament, which drew teams from other cities in our region of the country.

Teams from several states would compete, and major league scouts would attend. We were playing a strong team from Detroit, whose catcher (Ted Simmons) later became a St Louis Cardinals MLB all-star catcher. We had jumped ahead of the Detroit team and were fired up. I was playing third base when a foul ball was hit over my head toward an old retaining fence.

It would be close, but I had a chance to catch the ball for an out. As I stretched out my arm and when I barely caught the ball, I felt my waist hit the retaining fence, and felt my left leg go numb. When I turned to throw, both leg bones broke through the skin about six inches above my ankle, resulting in my lower leg being grotesquely at a 90-degree angle. I screamed and was in shock, as were my teammates and parents and sisters who were there. I later learned a couple of our starters took themselves out of the game, unable to continue. Our team was eliminated. Shattering my lower leg catching a foul ball in that tournament effectively ended my chance of ever playing as I previously did.

A Cincinnati Reds MLB scout at the game saw the sorrow of my parents and kindly gave my Dad a scouting card and said, "Your son is a disciplined and dedicated player, fill out and return the scouting card, and we'll follow him when he recovers."

This meant a lot to my parents and me and helped me get through a hard recovery and rehab process. I had surgery placing metal pins in my ankle and below my knee to stabilize my leg bones once a plaster cast was put around them, from my toes to my hip. The cast was on for 6 months, and my senior year as captain of my high school team was virtually wiped out. I cried when the cast was removed. My leg muscles had atrophied so much they looked more like my arm, rather than my other leg.

Rehab was hard and progress was slow. Starting with a terrible limp, I eventually got close to running normally. My doctor was amazed I got that far. He previously said I would never again run or play ball. I did play again, but I never again could pivot on my left leg as needed. I enjoyed playing summer-league baseball, and unsuccessfully (twice) tried to make the Ohio U team as a walk on.

I likely could have played at a smaller, private college, a couple of which expressed interest in granting a small scholarship. But I wanted the challenge of a bigger program, otherwise I would never know if I could play at that level. Another factor in my decision was that state supported colleges had far lower tuition and my parents worked hard to pay for my sisters and me to attend college.

While I was very disappointed at the time, looking back, unexpected, good things happened that likely would not have if not for the accident. I would not have gotten a medical draft deferment for my leg and likely would have gone to war in Vietnam. I would not have had as much time to study and earn the top spot in my business class, which helped get more job offers in several large cities. Kathleen and I may not have gotten married right after my graduation, and I avoided experiencing the horrible impacts of being in a war.

Now facing a dire cancer prognosis, I wondered, "Why can't unforeseen positive things also occur along with the seemingly impossible cancer hurdles in front of us?"

Cancer was going to get our best fight.

Kathleen completely supported me and she is the biggest reason I survived. I am blessed to have her love, understanding, tolerance, intelligence, and world-class caregiving. She gives me strength when I need it most. Without her, I would not have made it through several very tough spots that lay ahead.

Bob Kellermeyer Appointments

Kathleen and I liked Bob K the first time we met him. He projected an experienced, methodical, and confident style. We liked that he patiently answered our questions and quickly began building trust in him. When I asked about the long-term, he said, "Focus on one step at a time, don't jump ahead."

He replied to another key question, "Yes, I treat another myeloma patient who is in his fifth year of survival, and will ask his permission for you to contact him". We were grateful to talk with a survivor.

Bob explained he would start me on a chemotherapy and steroid mix that was his second choice, to see if it would reduce my urine protein level, the key indicator for my type of myeloma (Bence-Jones, or 'kappa light chain only'). Other myeloma types manifest in the blood. He explained the abnormal cells began in my marrow and leaked into my body and my urine. In my case, this caused bone damage where the abnormal cells were most concentrated.

My kidney function, as indicated by my serum creatinine, was impaired, and he advised me to drink a lot of fluid to help this function.

The array of monthly test results was overwhelming at the beginning. In time, we learned in my case two readings, urine monoclonal protein and serum creatinine, became my scorecard of how my treatments were doing. I started keeping track of both of these readings. I had to fill 24-hour urine bottles frequently to monitor the monoclonal (or abnormal) protein. My 24-collection showed how much I was drinking, and I used this to motivate me to stay well hydrated.

I began a regular paper pad of cancer notes, in chronological order. Capturing key information from appointments or tests helped me remember and form questions for follow up meetings. I used graph paper to plot monoclonal protein and serum creatinine and connect the points to show upward or downward trends.

Bob K advised, "Trends are more important than a single test results; don't put too much weight on a single result, see what the next test shows."

I continue to save my medical note pads, and draw line graphs when my disease is active. Years later, during an appointment with another hem/onc, my prior results were not showing on his computer screen, and he asked to see my records.

Bob K's other enduring advice was, "I only make one change at a time to treatments, to accurately see the result of that change."

Kathleen found an Italian article discussing bone thinning, such as mine from myeloma. Italian doctors found that giving monthly bisphosphonate intravenously in 2-hour treatments helped prevent further bone thinning or damage. She reviewed her findings with Bob K and asked if this may help me.

The doctor said he would read the article and let us know. That same evening, Bob K called and said that while he did not think this was being used in the US, he believed it was reasonable to do. I began taking the bone strengthening infusions in 1994. None of us are aware of any US myeloma patient who began taking these at that time.

Since then, other myeloma patients began taking this same treatment, and later another type of bisphosphonate taking less time to infuse. After doing more research, I decided to continue with the original 2-hour type, since I viewed my risk of a known side-effect risk to jaw bones as lower. Over the years, we changed the monthly treatments to less frequently.

Each myeloma case is different and affects patients differently. Some patients do not have bone effects, and some do not have their kidney functions affected, like I do. To me, Kathleen's bone thinning research and question of our doctor is an example of partnering with our doctor—a strategy we continue to find useful.

Starting with Bob K's second choice meant we would have his first choice if the first one failed to reduce my protein level. We liked this reasoning since we were saving something for later if we need it. It allowed us to sleep a bit easier, since Kathleen's research indicated myeloma treatments had not changed much in about 4 decades. No new myeloma drugs were on the scene in 1992.

Informing Family and Friends

We did not want to delay sharing my cancer diagnosis with our sons, my parents and two sisters, and Kathleen's family. But we thought it would be easier for them (especially for my Dad) to give the bad news after we met with Bob Kellermeyer and understood specifics. We knew our families would have questions, and our answers had to be honest and as encouraging as possible. We agreed that we would not withhold bad news.

After my first cycle of chemo, we met with our families in person to break the news. We scheduled a college visit on their upcoming Parents Weekend to tell Jim and Bob that I had cancer. We borrowed an approach of saying myeloma has no cure, *yet*. Years before I was diagnosed, a friend had buttons made with "yet" on them which reinforced his point that a sales goal may not be met. He preferred to say the goal has not been achieved, yet. Our sons even gave me a hat with "yet" on it and my administrative assistant, Marilyn Willis had stickers made with "yet" as well.

Jim and Bob took the news as well as could be expected. They had planned weekend events, and we followed through with the bad news on our minds. They are both strong, and we're grateful they were at the same college for one another. We promised to tell them good, and bad news, which seemed to help a little.

They offered their help with anything we needed. It was a long drive home. I recall being thankful we started our family as soon as we married. I had two decades of being with our sons. Had we waited to have children; I would have had less time until this deadly blood cancer hit.

We told the rest of our families at meals together. They were relieved to see I was able to eat normally, and noticed my face was rounder than normal, which was from the steroid I was taking. Bob K referred to this as being "moon faced."

In terms of our friends and co-workers, our initial judgment was to keep my diagnosis as private as we could. At the time, my thinking was this would help allow us to be as normal as possible and not let cancer invade our lives any more than necessary.

Ultimately, I was wrong to withhold the news. After a while, we changed and opened up with friends and colleagues. We quickly realized it helped to have more people to support us and it allowed us to let go some of our feelings. Everyone understood and offered to help. My EY colleagues stepped in for me when I needed to be at medical appointments.

Gaining Confidence

We divided cancer responsibilities at home. Kathleen managed my health insurance matters, including difficult discussions with an insurance provider denying coverage on a required procedure. EY was key to helping out with this and supporting us at every turn. Kathleen took control of my scheduled medication, making my job easy taking pills as requested. My job was to manage my health, comply with my doctor's orders, and take care of myself. I exercised daily in some form believing it would make me stronger to withstand the damage from chemotherapy.

Steroids were preventing me from sleeping normally, but they were part of the mix needed to fight the myeloma. I had to deal with it. At times steroids made my thinking and behavior chaotic. Our sons gave me another hat, this one with "Captain Chaos" on it. We got through it together.

After a couple months, the initial treatment plan was not working, and my doctor decided it was time to start the chemo mix he thought was our best weapon. It involved wearing a small pump under my shirt with a tube to a port in my chest to receive the drugs continuously. I was able to go to work with this set-up without others being aware of it. In that era, men in our office wore suits, and the pump and tube were hidden under my shirt and suit coat.

After one treatment of the new chemo mix, my urine protein began to decline as we prayed it would. A trend began, and I soon was in complete remission, or zero monoclonal protein and no new bone pain. My broken ribs felt better. We were very grateful. But we did not celebrate. We knew myeloma would come back, the question was how long would I stay in remission.

Our roller-coaster ride had begun.

The Transplant Decision

Before our initial appointment with Bob K, Kathleen and I composed a short fax to other hem/oncs around the country who specialized in multiple myeloma. Kathleen's library research surfaced a handful of doctors who published several myeloma treatment and research articles. In 1992, since priority was given to a fax, we faxed these doctors, briefly outlining my diagnosis and who was going to treat me. I asked, "If you were in my shoes, would you proceed with this plan, or go somewhere else?"

Each doctor quickly agreed we were in good hands with Bob K, most of whom knew Bob from meetings. The additional endorsements added to our confidence level that we were not missing something.

After gaining complete remission from the chemo treatments, Bob K discussed a decision we now had to make. Autologous stem cell bone marrow transplants (auto transplants) were starting to be used with the goal of prolonging remission for patients with multiple myeloma. He explained that I qualified to have stem cells harvested from my blood, since tests showed no monoclonal protein. Since then, tests have advanced to detect even slighter amounts of this abnormal protein. As long as I stayed in remission, UH would admit me for one of their first myeloma auto transplants. Other cancer centers were successfully completing the transplants, having learned how to minimize the risk of a patient dying from the procedure. UH was the first in Ohio to do adult transplants.

We felt we needed to decide soon, since no one knew how long my remission would last. Kathleen led our research on the pros and cons of doing a transplant, aided by Bob K's guidance and article references. We concluded that doing a transplant would be like buying insurance. It would give us comfort that we did all we could to keep myeloma in remission. We could not find any clinical trials showing I would live longer with or without a transplant, but many believe it may prolong a remission. Since our doctor was recommending it, and our research supported its being a good strategy, we decided to do the transplant immediately. Basically, deciding to kick it while it's down.

A large insurance provider of my firm's sponsored medical insurance choices initially denied us coverage of this procedure, claiming it was "Experimental and not in the patient's best interest". They adamantly argued against covering the transplant, despite our respected doctor's opinion that it was my best course of action. Kathleen was terribly upset with the insurance company denying the coverage. Frustrating calls with the insurance company added to her already high stress level. Dr. Kellermeyer asked Kathleen to assist him with more research to bolster his original letter that the transplant was necessary for me. A third letter was written, but we were still being denied. Kathleen told the insurance company we may talk to a lawyer (do not get her riled up).

After discussing our dilemma with EY and following their recommendations, a second, firm-sponsored insurance provider quickly agreed it was reasonable to do and they covered my transplant. Without my firm's support, the transplant would not have been covered. I was grateful to have spent my entire 24 years working hard for EY. It is impossible to place a value on our firm's support when I needed it the most.

Certain memories stand out in my transplant. The first step was scheduling two days of electrophoresis for harvesting stem cells from my blood. This was preceded by injections to boost the white count and therefore the stem cells. An IV in one arm took my blood out, ran it through a machine, and returned my blood in an IV in the other arm. The machine separated my stem cells from my other blood components and when later injected back into me through a port in my chest, the stem cells make their way in to repopulate the bone marrow. Each day's batch of stem cells were frozen. When enough cells were gathered, I was ready to be admitted to the transplant floor. Other tests were done to ensure I was otherwise in good health.

Unfortunately, shortly before the harvesting of stem cells was to begin, I developed a fever, which continued to rise. Kathleen called Bob K, who was concerned, and said to meet him at UH in general admitting right away. He seemed more concerned than we had seen him in the past. He ordered the admissions personnel to bypass the normal paperwork and get me into a hospital bed immediately. They diagnosed a bacterial infection, and the infectious disease doctor began daily cultures and tried different drugs to control the infection.

Cultures take days to grow bacteria, and it took quite a while to find the drug that worked. I recall being anxious to begin the transplant. Bob K was again helpful by advising that stress can adversely affect cancer patients.

Autologous Stem Cell Transplant

Signing my first lengthy consent was sobering. The consent detailed each possible transplant risk, including the low risk of dying. I agreed to do the transplant in a clinical trial setting, since trials capture and summarize patient results needed to advance treatments.

We learned there is another 'time zone 'in our country, which we now call "hospital time." Naively, I expected hospital doctors to appear at the time given to me or have someone inform me they were running late. This was the culture I experienced in my work and I expected the same in a hospital setting. I became educated that medical systems just operate differently, but only after a heated exchange with the UH transplant doctor. Over time, we developed a reasonably good working relationship. We even took the doctor and his wife to a Cleveland Indians game since he and I shared a common interest in baseball.

Entering UH's bone marrow transplant floor was different than being on other hospital floors and it was very restricted. To limit risk of infections, transplant visitors were limited, and at times had to wear face masks in the rooms and wash/disinfect their hands frequently. Plants were not allowed. I asked my family and friends if they would donate blood platelets, which I would need when mine were intentionally wiped out by heavy doses of chemotherapy. I was touched when my family, friends, co-workers, and clients donated their platelets to help. A co-worker and one client executive donated despite their fear of needles and the sight of blood.

I was hospitalized for two weeks, and Kathleen was with me each day. We advised our sons to stay at Miami University. Bob K visited often and each visit was meaningful. Their visits were the highlights of my day. There was no email or internet in those days to occupy the time.

My goal was to be out of my bed and walking around as much as possible, convinced that some form of daily exercise would help me better withstand the heavy doses of chemotherapy needed. UH's transplant nurses in 1993 were used to transplant patients staying in bed most of the day. This has changed over time, in part due to patients who were determined to be active.

In addition to heavy doses of chemotherapy, my protocol included two days, twice a day of full-body radiation. It was unsettling to be locked in a metal vault-like room for each treatment. The radiation and chemotherapy combination soon wiped out my bone marrow and immune system. They also produced nausea and fatigue, growing worse each day until I was completely uncomfortable, in or out of bed. Morphine was dripped into my IV to make me comfortable. I quickly lobbied for the morphine to be gradually tapered and then stopped.

Some days, all I could do physically was make myself sit up in bed. Next, I made myself stand next to the bed for as long as I could. When I felt strong enough, I pulled my IV pole and pumps around the transplant floor, much to the dismay of several nurses. Much has changed today on the transplant floor of University Hospital's Seidman Cancer Center which has an exercise room and wider hallways for patients to walk.

After a while, my daily key blood test became my ANC (absolute neutrophil count). When it declined to near zero, it was time to unfreeze my stem cells collected earlier and inject them into my blood stream through a port in my chest. Watching the nurse walk across my room with these cells seemed like science fiction. The bag of cells she was holding was my only way to survive. It was scary and required the ultimate trust.

After receiving my cells, and a few more days of zero ANC, my counts slowly started to increase. I was very relieved to witness the plan working. A reading of 50 ANC was needed to be discharged, and Jim's college graduation was coming up soon. Kathleen let him know I would still be hospitalized, and he understood, but we were all disappointed. On the Wednesday before his commencement, I asked my nurse if she could please start expediting the paperwork and other discharge requirements. I hoped that my ANC would rise to 50 by Friday. It was a long shot, but it was possible, and nurse Tina Shin compassionately helped us.

After Discharge

Fortunately, my ANC hit 50 on Friday and I was discharged the next morning. With the doctor's approval, Kathleen drove us a few hundred miles to Jim's commencement. I recall ordering from the children's menu when we stopped for a meal since I could not eat an adult sized entree.

Jim had not picked up his graduation cap and gown since he was sure we could not attend. His disbelief equaled ours when we saw him. He scrambled and got a cap and gown in time to go through the commencement. It seemed impossible to believe, considering where we had been just a few days before. College graduations are emotional for parents and we treasured being at Jim's even more given the circumstances. It was remarkable from one Sunday to the next, I went from being out of it on morphine to sitting at our older son's graduation.

Kathleen recalls my transplant time being shorter than any other UH patient, and significantly shorter than they told us to plan on being there. I was told to allow 4 to 6 weeks and amazingly was out in two weeks! It was great returning home, recuperating, and trying to return to normal after a whirlwind experience. Within a month, I was back at work, feeling good, and serving my client assignments. However, Kathleen was not herself. She was stressed-out, with nothing more for her to do for my cancer and treatment, except worry about when the myeloma would return.

That all changed one day after I drove to work and called her an hour later and said, "I am fine, but the car is not. A pink Buick ran a red light and crashed into the driver's side of our car. The pink Buick pushed me and our car into the one next to me."

Kathleen was very upset and screamed, "How *could you* get in a car accident after all we've been through!"

I was silent; she paused and then realized it could happen to anyone. She tells people this helped ease her stress and worry over cancer. None of us know when our days are over, cancer or not. And, she likes to add, "Watch out for those pink Buicks."

We were again thrilled to attend Bob's college graduation in three years and still later to be at his wedding to Stacey. Bob adopted Stacey's young daughter, Jillian, our first grandchild. We were happy when they moved back to our neighborhood from Chicago. Life was good.

I remained in remission for almost 6 years and Bob K did not suggest any maintenance drugs. I saw him at about 3 or 6-month intervals to monitor my myeloma remission by dropping off 24-hour urine, have blood drawn, and discuss our questions. Kathleen continued to read about myeloma and related subjects as we knew we needed to keep our eyes on the horizon regarding new myeloma treatments.

My medical focus was on doing another auto transplant, since I was aware other myeloma patients had extended their remissions by doing more than one. No new myeloma drugs were yet on the scene. Bob K was supportive, but I would need to convince the UH transplant leader who had done my first one to proceed with a second transplant. Unfortunately, there was concern whether stem cells could be harvested again from me since I had already been through one transplant with radiation and heavy chemo. All of the stem cells collected were used in that first transplant.

Second Auto

When the monoclonal protein began to rise, the transplant doctor agreed to meet with me and explain his position. He felt it was unlikely I could produce enough stem cells to harvest for a second auto transplant, because of the radiation and drugs needed for my first one.

I pressed him by asking, "What do I need to do to have you try another transplant?"

He didn't seem accustomed to being questioned by a patient, but I was doing all I could do to survive. I recall he reluctantly responded, "If you are willing to visit Phil Greipp (Phil G) at the Mayo Clinic, and if they would do another transplant , then we will do it here."

Kathleen and I traveled to Rochester MN., where I was examined and tested before meeting with a transplant doctor and then Phil G. At this point, my note taking ability gave way to asking permission to use a tape recorder to get the most from key doctor visits. Like other doctors, Phil G was happy to allow me to use a recorder. He was a great guy we ended up seeing a second time a few years later and staying in touch with until he passed away. He knew my UH transplant doctor from meetings they attended, and they respected one another.

Phil G concluded that he agreed doing a second auto transplant in my situation was reasonable, and Mayo would be happy to do it. He added, "You are in good hands with your UH transplant doctor and being close to your home has advantages for both of you."

Kathleen and I found that using a tape recorder helps us be more engaged in doctor visits and accurately understand what was said after the fact. Once we were home from a doctor visit, I would transcribe the tape contents to my chronological medical note pad. On one drive home, Kathleen and I were discussing what the doctor said that day and we had a disagreement. I thought the doctor said one thing, and Kathleen thought something different. To our surprise, when I transcribed the conversation, we were both wrong! The doctor had said something different than either of us recalled. We have learned that being under stress can cause misunderstandings.

We returned home from Rochester, MN and met with the transplant doctor who was now willing to move forward with my second auto transplant. Persistence had paid off for us. It's another example of teamwork with doctors, and an example of the value of second opinions for key decisions. Maintaining contact with these out-of-town specialists has proven very valuable.

In my second transplant, Bob K used the same drug mix used to reduce monoclonal protein in advance of admitting me. My second auto transplant experience was like the first, except there was no full body radiation. I again agreed to participate in a clinical trial as part of the transplant. Advances in certain new drugs, including a drug that boosted production of more stem cells and no radiation made this one seem easier than the first. But it was still time out of our lives for hospitalization, more stress on Kathleen, our sons, and other family. During that time, it lifted my spirits to have family, friends and our family doctor, Kevin Geraci dropping in to visit.

The second transplant produced a remission lasting almost 2 years. Unlike the first remission, some abnormal protein and low blood counts occasionally appeared, causing us to worry about our next option.

The UH medical team approved of Kathleen giving me periodic shots of a white cell booster without having to go to the hospital.

No new myeloma drugs were yet available, except thalidomide. It was an old drug once used as a pregnancy morning sickness sedative with tragic results, however it was showing some promise for myeloma patients. I agreed with Bob K it was worth a try since nothing else was available. It was not helpful, and it caused slight neuropathy in my hands and bottom of my feet, which fortunately do not really bother me.

Mini Allo Idea

Bob K wisely suggested my two sisters, Becki and Denyse, be tested to see if their stem cells matched mine. The UH transplant doctor could do a mini, or low intensity, allogeneic (mini allo) stem cell transplant if either sister's cells matched mine. Both Becki and Denyse were eager to help and fortunately Becki was a match. I am grateful for both my sisters.

Driving 70 miles to donate her stem cells was hard for Becki who fears needles and the sight of blood. Kathleen helped Becki get through her UH stem cell harvesting session by providing comfort and distracting Becki from the IVs in both arms for hours at a time. To avoid Becki watching the blood flow out and back into her arms, Kathleen draped cloths over the tubes to keep the blood out of sight. I am forever grateful for Becki's selflessness and kindness. It helped me to remain hopeful, and ultimately stay alive.

Bob K contacted Phil G at the Mayo Clinic and they discussed the possibility of me having a mini-allo transplant. Phil G asked us to visit him, which we did, and he agreed the mini allo was reasonable in my case. I asked him if there were other myeloma drugs in clinical trials that may help me. He said yes there was one called PS341 showing good preliminary results for sick myeloma patients like me.

He said if I got in trouble, "Ypu should run, not walk, to try to get into a PS341 clinical trial."

Kathleen, Bob K and I discussed the pros and cons of doing the mini allo or trying to get in the PS341 that Phil G had discussed with us. It was difficult to decide.

Bob K was friends with another top-notch transplant oncology specialist, Tom Spitzer, at Massachusetts General Hospital in Boston. Tom trained at UH under the well-known UH transplant doctor. Bob K spoke highly of Tom, who had had already performed several successful mini allos for myeloma patients. Bob encouraged us to visit Tom to help us decide between the mini allo or possibly finding an opening in the PS341 trial.

Tom was very gracious with us, showing us the transplant floor and describing his protocol, which I learned is proprietary information. He said the UH transplant doctor, would be an equally good choice, but he was happy to do it if we decided Tom was our preference. We would have to relocate to Boston if we chose Tom. His opinion helped our confidence with doing the mini allo at UH rather than relocating for months. We are still in contact with Tom.

The myeloma was growing quickly while I was going through tests before being admitted for the mini allo. After an X-ray, Bob K informed me my high protein level had caused an egg-shaped hole near the top of my left arm, making it at risk for breaking. I had to have a 10-inch metal plate surgically fastened to the arm bone to stabilize it before doing a transplant. It would have been big trouble for my arm to break while doing a transplant and with no immune system.

We worried about my quickly increasing disease level with no way to slow it. After my arm surgery was done the transplant doctor told us my high level of abnormal protein means the planned mini allow was unlikely to be enough to combat the myeloma. However, he would do the transplant since Becki's cells were harvested, and I was admitted for the mini allo. I am grateful he agreed to go forward.

Bob K, Phil G, Tom S and the UH transplant doctor were important to our decision agreement to go forward.

Mini Allo

I was admitted to the transplant floor. At one point during the mini-allo, my white blood count became too low, and the UH team decided to give me white cells to boost mine, which I was told is unusual. Becki's white cells were also needed, and she again donated and helped tremendously. Some of her white cells were saved for possible direct leukocyte infusion (DLI), should it be necessary, which it was.

My bone marrow grew back, only this time it was Becki's immune system in me, rather than mine; Kathleen later joked, "Jim was a lot more fun to shop with after receiving his sister's stem cells."

Kathleen's a funny girl. Admittedly, I did buy some new shoes I had been putting off for a while.

I was discharged and told to stay quarantined in our house for 100 days while I recovered. My diet was restricted due to my low immune system. Although it was stressful for her, Kathleen served as a home nurse and giving me certain shots. She did a great job caring for me and calling one of my doctors or nurses for any advice needed.

'Go to Hospice'

After 100 days, my transplant was fine, but the abnormal protein was again increasing, now at a dangerous level. I received DLI as a possible way to control myeloma, but nothing would slow down the growing abnormal protein. My kidney function was impaired, my legs were swelling, I had a 105-degree fever, and was unable to eat much. Additionally, I needed daily blood transfusions to stay alive.

I recall the transplant doctor telling me, "Jim you need to go to a hospice; there is nothing else left to help."

I replied, "What about the PS341 clinical trial Phil G told us was showing promising results, on a preliminary basis, for sick myeloma patients like me?"

Then I recall he said, "I know all about that trial, and there are no PS341 clinical trials open anywhere that can help you in time. You would be wasting your time to even try."

I replied, "I am going to try."

I recall he abruptly left the room seemingly frustrated that we were not following his advice to go to a hospice.

I thought about this exchange and was incredulous. How could the transplant doctor think I would be *wasting my time* when he just advised me to go to a hospice? We would not lose hope, and we would not give up.

While the mini allo did not produce a remission, perhaps these three additional months were key to Dana Farber's having an opening that likely was not there when I started the mini allo. My view is to stay in the game each day I can. The future may have a new drug or procedure. It is unlikely to come from behind in the bottom of the ninth inning, or with only seconds left on the clock, but it *can* happen.

Never give up.

All Hope Not Lost

I contacted Phil G and asked him if he would recommend some hospitals and doctors who may have a PS341 opening. He gave me a few and added there was nothing anyone could do to increase my chances of being admitted, but it was worth my asking.

I was still actively working at EY, years away from retirement age. I left phone messages with each doctor Phil G had recommended, including a doctor at the start-up pharma development company, Millennium Pharmaceutical, that developed PS341. While the drug company was not itself conducting clinical trials, it worked with hospitals whose myeloma doctors were conducting trials. He gave me another name to contact.

I was praying for a return call from any of these doctors. As a practicing CPA, I was analytic, and summarized my myeloma recent test results into handwritten graphs showing my trends and history. I wanted to answer any questions the best way I could when a doctor called back. On a Friday I will not forget; I was in my office and the phone rang.

A young sounding doctor with a British accent said, "Hello Jim, Paul Richardson here at Dana Farber in Boston. I know a little about your case, and I only have two questions."

I'm thinking with only two questions, they may be difficult. He asked, "First, are you and your wife willing to relocate from the Cleveland area to the Boston area for nine months? "

I quickly replied, "Yes". It was an easy decision. We had just been told I should go to a hospice, and this doctor was talking about me being alive for nine more months.

"Second, how soon can you two get to Boston?" He asked. I said, "We can be there tomorrow."

He said, "Tomorrow is Saturday, and Monday would be fine." I was thrilled and told Kathleen the news. She let our sons and other family know. I went home and packed for nine months. I noticed Kathleen seemed to be only packing enough for a few days. I disregarded it, knowing my thinking was likely impacted by my high fever. My sister Denyse, and her husband, Charlie dropped us off at the airport. When she said goodbye, she hugged me and seemed to be saying good-bye forever, not for just nine months. Again, I put it out of my mind, thinking it was my fever causing these thoughts.

Dana Farber

We arrived at our hotel near Dana Farber. I was feeling awful and went to bed. Kathleen later told me my fever reached 105, my legs were swelling up and I looked terrible. She was unsure I would live through the night and make it to Dana Farber the next day. She called the myeloma cancer center's emergency night phone number.

Ken Anderson, the leader of Dana's myeloma group was on duty handling after hour emergencies that night. Kathleen's earlier research included myeloma articles he had written. Ken instructed her how to get me through the night, and gave her some comfort by agreeing the myeloma could be causing my high temperature, leg swelling, and sick feeling.

He added, "Mrs. Bond, did anyone tell you that Jim is the seventh patient admitted to our PS341 trial, and his study number is 007? I think that is good karma."

He was correct. After overcoming some obstacles, it was good karma.

My first hurdle was that my clinical doctor, Paul Richardson (Paul R), who had called me earlier, had to admit me into Dana's affiliated hospital near them. My tenuous condition needed to improve before I could meet the criteria of entering the PS341 trial as an outpatient, not as a hospitalized patient.

The clinical trial made this necessary, but it presented a life-threatening dilemma. Kathleen and I knew the high myeloma level caused my condition, yet the only hope we had to control the myeloma was to be discharged and qualify to be admitted to the trial as an outpatient.

I was in no condition to effectively plead our case to the young Dana myeloma doctor, (Rob Schlossman), attending me in the hospital. But Kathleen was great and convinced him what she was saying was reasonable and that she understood myeloma well. Rob S saved my life by taking a chance.

He told us, "I am discharging you to your hotel so that you can come into Dana as an outpatient and begin PS341 treatments."

My clinical trial nurse, Debby Doss (Debby D) did us a similar big favor helping us into the trial. Earlier, when my kidney function test results just barely met the admission criteria, I recall she advised me not to have any further such tests. We suspected my kidneys likely were declining, and another test could disqualify me from admission to the trial. Debbie also told us we could not be admitted in the trial until the required time elapsed from my last UH treatment. Clinical trials are necessarily rigid in admission criteria, to help get FDA approval.

We remain in contact with Debby D and Rob S both of whom retired from Dana years later. We will not forget their compassion.

Within 2 weeks from entering the trial (four treatments) I was feeling much better. I was able to eat some soft foods for the first time in a while. My leg swelling improved and my high temperature was gone. Kathleen could see the PS341 experimental drug was working.

This was confirmed when Debby D sought us out in the patient waiting room, waving a sheet of my test results and smiling. She excitedly said, "Jim, we're not aware of such a dramatic response to PS341. Your very high level of abnormal protein is nearly gone in only two weeks!"

She cautioned us that these results needed to be confirmed in a week or two. Like Bob K, she believed one test result is not definitive by itself. We need to see a trend, which the next test confirmed.

Ninety-nine percent of my very high abnormal protein had vanished in 2 weeks!

By the end of the trial, I was back in remission. To us, this experimental drug was a miracle. Our close call demonstrated how quickly things can change, and to never give up. The drug was approved in record time and has helped many other patients around the world. It is called Velcade, the first of its class of proteasome inhibitors.

Sandy Cunningham

The first day Kathleen and I were in Dana Farber's infusion room a volunteer came with his food cart and offered a sandwich for lunch. I explained I was too sick to eat. Ingersoll (Sandy) Cunningham persisted and offered fruit or crackers, but I could not eat. It was Memorial Day weekend, and Sandy was wearing a bow tie (his trademark) and a straw hat. Both were decorated in red, white, and blue.

I asked about his bow tie and hat and asked if he was a veteran. This led to a good discussion of his WWII experience, a subject I enjoy learning about. Sandy told me he was a retired banker, and long-time Dana volunteer, as was his wife Sheila, who founded and led 'The Friends of Dana Farber' program. He was more interested in our story, and he intently listened, and then asked, "Well, where are you and Kathleen staying for the remainder of your nine months in the Boston area?"

I explained we were looking for an apartment downtown and afterwards look for something to rent in the suburbs. Without hesitation he replied, "You two can have our house in a suburb, since we are going to spend the summer at our family house on the Cape. But you'll have to pay the weekly housekeeper and water the lawn."

I was overwhelmed by his kindness. After a first meeting and a short conversation, Sandy offered us the use of his house for almost no cost. Who does that? We consider ourselves fairly nice people, but I doubt we would have done the same if our roles were reversed. Sandy cautioned, "Now, we'll both have to check with our wives to see if they agree with you and me. And, Sheila will want to meet you, and Kathleen will want to see our house."

Kathleen was amazed and a little tentative until she and I further discussed this with Sandy and Sheila. Sandy drove Kathleen out to see their suburban home, and we could not believe our luck, or good karma. We enjoyed living in their home and became lasting friends with Sandy. Sheila passed away from cancer months later; Sandy remarried to their life-long friend who lost her husband. We were with them on their fifth wedding anniversary when they were in their eighties. We saw them frequently when we were on vacation near their summer home.

Over the years, Sandy was like a second father to me, and we were sorry to see him depart at ninety-six. A memorial card by his daughter Jen perfectly described her father's approach to life as follows:

"Life is short, we don't have much time; be quick to love and be kind."

More than ever, I strive to have these qualities.

Our cancer experience also showed us that each person with myeloma is unique. Many other sick myeloma patients across the country were in separate arms of PS341. To my knowledge, no other response was as dramatic as mine. We realized we are very fortunate.

Velcade Background

The start-up pharma company that developed Velcade invited Paul R and us to a company celebration on the day they gained FDA approval. We were honored to share the stage with Paul R and express our thanks to the company's life-saving employees. I thanked Julian Adams; the company's lead scientist who tenaciously pushed for the development of the experimental drug that saved my life.

At the company meeting, I met Julian, who stopped me when I tried to fill in some of my story and said, "Jim, since your response, I have learned more about you than you know."

Julian's picture appeared on a prominent magazine after Velcade was approved. I later learned the start-up company nearly had to stop the PS341 trial before I received the drug. Company funders were not seeing the results they hoped for and were hesitant to make additional funds available to continue the trial. But my dramatic response and other responses came just in time to change their minds and continue funding for the trial. Thousands of myeloma patients worldwide have used this valuable myeloma option. I remain in contact with Julian. Takeda Pharmaceutical purchased the startup company, Millennium Pharmaceutical, that discovered Velcade and we also keep in contact with Takeda.

After starting as a door-to-door fundraiser, Kathleen became a top volunteer leader for American Cancer Society (ACS). Kathleen learned that three researchers funded by the ACS were the team that opened the pathway that enabled Julian's team to advance the research and discover Velcade. The three scientists received a Nobel Prize for their fundamental research. They are among 49 recipients of a Nobel Prize that were funded early in their careers by the ACS. No other non-governmental cancer group has funded nearly as many Nobel winners. When the ACS leaders learned that I was saved by such research, they made a video telling our story which was posted on YouTube.

Life after Velcade

While completing the nine-month clinical trial and living in the Boston area, our son Jim and his fiancé, Emilee planned a Labor Day Weekend wedding. Paul assured me when I began the clinical trial that I would be able to attend their wedding in Chicago. His optimism inspired me, but we had real doubts with my situation when we first arrived at Dana. We were thrilled and grateful to attend their wedding.

While we were in Boston, my Dad's different forms of cancer hospitalized him, and we had our last conversation on the phone, since a fever sadly prevented me from traveling home to be with him, his second wife, Pat, my sisters, and the rest of our family.

A few years earlier we were grateful and thrilled to attend Bob's college graduation. A couple years after the Velcade trail we were again grateful to attend Bob's wedding to Stacey in Chicago, where they both lived with Stacey's daughter, Jillian. Bob adopted Jillian and we were delighted to welcome our first grandchild. Jim and Emilee had two sons, Dayton and Wade who equally bless us.

Our sons' marriages and eventually having three grandchildren seemed like impossible dreams when I was diagnosed.

As expected, myeloma returned in a about a year after Velcade ended. But the monoclonal protein did not rise very high, unlike before Velcade. The slight amount of abnormal protein was not rising rapidly, and I contacted Paul. He asked if I would do him a favor and enter another clinical trial he was helping to lead at Dana. I was happy to help Paul after he and his team saved my life. We returned to Boston and I entered another experimental drug clinical trial. It did not reduce the abnormal protein, but my abnormal protein was fairly low and stable. We remained calm and confident in Paul, who then recommended another clinical trial of an experimental drug showing good preliminary results with other patients.

We agreed and needed to relocate to Boston for about three months. The drug was effective in reducing my small amount of abnormal protein to zero. While living in the Boston area, I needed to have cataracts removed, a known risk of the full body radiation received during my first transplant.

Back in remission, we returned to our Cleveland area home. We attended a UH transplant survivors' event. I recall the UH transplant doctor congratulating me on our decision to enter the PS341 clinical trial. I also recall his telling me he suspected my dramatic response to PS341 may also have been due to the mini allo so close to entering the trial.

Following Paul's advice to take a lower dose of the experimental drug as maintenance. The FDA approved that myeloma drug while I was doing the trial, and it has helped many patients.

I continued a low dose of that drug as a maintenance drug, along with a low steroid dose, to hopefully prolong my remission. I was having a lot of trouble walking due to pain in my right thigh. I thought maybe I pulled a muscle, but x-rays showed the top of my hip bone had eroded away causing my pain. The orthopedic surgeon explained this is a risk of cancer patients who need to take steroids over a long period. He inserted a metal rod in the bone and replaced that hip with a metal ball and socket. My continues to be good, which annual x-rays confirm.

After hearing that such bone erosion is a risk from steroids, I began to question the need to use a steroid with my current maintenance drug and other myeloma drugs. I discussed my risk with myeloma doctors, and we agreed to stop my steroids which many protocols typically contain. We were learning that for me, myeloma was becoming a marathon, not a sprint. I will agree to use steroids when absolutely necessary. I believe they are a powerful weapon against myeloma.

Kathleen spotted a suspicious spot on my back that the UH dermatologist diagnosed as skin cancer, but thankfully not melanoma that took my sister, Janell. He removed the skin cancer and examined all my skin for others. He explained that having even one stem cell transplant causes high risk of skin cancer, due to immune system effects. The dermatologist examines my skin multiple times a year, regardless of whether I spot something suspicious. Almost every time, a skin cancer is found and removed.

Kathleen's Big Idea

After our successful Boston experiences, Kathleen and I discussed our good fortune being able to work remotely on a laptop and to have resources that allowed us to relocate from Cleveland twice.

She agreed and reminded me, "This is why the ACS operates over 30 Hope Lodges around the country, so that patients and caregivers needing to leave their home town can do so for free lodging."

I asked if there is a way to raise awareness to ACS Hope Lodges. She explained the ACS does not use donor funds to advertise its Hope Lodges. Late one night, Kathleen woke me from sleeping and said she had an idea for raising awareness and funds for Hope Lodges. I listened as she excitedly explained she could create a cycling event in Ohio in which people would ride from Cleveland to Cincinnati at the other end of the state. Both cities had Hope Lodges. Riders would raise money in support of their ride. It would not be a race; it would be a bike tour on bike paths and country roads. College dorms could house riders and supporting ACS staff and volunteers.

I said, "Honey, that's a good idea except neither of us cycles, or even owns a bike." She replied, "Not a problem; I will work with ACS Ohio management and staff and work that out."

ACS leaders knew and respected Kathleen from her years volunteering on other projects, including her successful leadership of significant fundraising for the Cleveland Hope Lodge, where she formed and led a volunteer advisory board.

I watched as she threw herself into overcoming challenges that her 328-mile bike ride presented, especially difficult for her with no cycling experience. She had done this before when she volunteered and became a junior high girls basketball team coach with no basketball background of her own. She did research and teamed with people who had basketball experience.

ACS Pan Ohio Hope Ride

ACS leadership introduced her to another volunteer, Dennis Hoffer, who had a different fundraising idea, which puzzled Kathleen until she learned Dennis was also an experienced cyclist. He had recently ridden his bike across Vietnam. He and Kathleen were a great team as co-leaders for over a decade, both committed to helping people with cancer. His cycling enthusiasm was matched with her passionate fundraising.

Together, they decided on a 4-day, 328-mile bike tour, with riders and others staying in selected college dorms along the way. Kathleen visited a AAA office and studied country roads and bike paths between Cleveland and Cincinnati. Dennis cycled many possible routes to decide on the safest ones for our riders. It became the ACS Pan Ohio Hope Ride (POHR).

College dorms were selected, and Penske Trucking kindly donated the use of trucks to haul the luggage of riders to the next stop and bring bikes back to the start when the ride ended. Penske continues to donate its trucks.

For two years on the sidelines, I watched her passionately turn her bike ride idea into a reality. I had to do more to support her hard work. I consulted with Dennis, bought a road bike, and followed his training advice.

ACS POHR Karma

The ACS Pan Ohio Hope Ride was set to begin in 2007 with about 50 of us riders. Shortly before the start in Cleveland, some of our family were participating in a myeloma fund raising event, including Bob and his family who had moved to Cleveland.

A local TV reporter who knew my medical history, asked our son, "Bob, do you really believe your dad, a non-cyclist who has some cancer side effects can ride his bike 328 miles in 4 days to Cincinnati?"

When we got home, I heard Bob's answer on TV. He said, "I don't know if Dad will make it all the way to the finish, but I will say this about my dad. When he says he'll do something, he will do it."

Bob's comments meant a lot to me, and still do. I felt motivated to do more than just riding a few hours daily. With our older son, Jim, and Bob's wife, Stacey, riding with me along the country roads and bike trails, I cycled all 4 days, all 328 miles.

I did the same each of the following 11 years, until it made more sense to ride fewer than 328 miles. I continue to fundraise for the ACS POHR.

I've been asked if it was hard for me to ride my bike 328 miles in 4 days. I reply, "Yes, long distance cycling is very hard, but not as hard as dealing with an incurable blood cancer, like myeloma."

 Daily exercise is one of the key reasons I survived many years and difficult treatments. Training for the POHR each year provided my exercise in the spring. At other times, exercise included doing all our yard work, walking the neighborhood or a treadmill and playing golf.

Kathleen was our co-leader throughout, and her idea has raised awareness not only to Hope Lodges, but also awareness to ACS research, their 24-7 support line, and other patient services. In its first 13 years, POHR riders and volunteers raised $10.5 million. POHR.org has details. POHR's rider return rate each year is unheard of for a multi-day cycling event. About 300 riders cycle each year. Our riders and volunteers look forward to being together each July for four days to help people with cancer and safely have fun cycling.

Our son, Jim, was concerned I would not be able to cycle the 2013 POHR. He touched me and many others by riding his bike alone an extra 300+ miles from Chicago to Cleveland to substitute for the POHR miles he thought I would miss. He did this right before the start of the POHR.

Jim's selflessness reminded me when he touched me years earlier when we were playing golf. As we walked down the fairway, I recall saying to Jim, "Now that you've graduated from college and are leaving home for your first job, I guess my days of offering advice are over."

I recall Jim responded, "Dad nothing could be further from the truth. I will value your advice forever."

When I was diagnosed, I thought there would be no more memories like this with Jim. But these memories have continued.

For my 60th birthday Jim took me to Scotland to golf with him on their legendary courses, including Carnoustie. I will never forget sinking a 40-foot putt across an undulating green with Jim on that trip.

Plasmacytoma

After more time passed, my abnormal protein began to rise, and Paul recommended increasing the dose of maintenance drug which I did. I also developed what was thought to be a cyst on the back of my head. The surgeon was starting to remove it, when he quickly stopped and said, "This is not a cyst; it is something else. You need to see your oncologist."

It was a plasmacytoma caused by the myeloma. Paul explained myeloma can do this, even though it had not happened to me before. I had several days of radiation treatments to eliminate the plasmacytoma. These were uncomfortable because my head had to be immobilized so that the radiation beam would only hit the right spot and not damage other head areas. A wet piece of fiberglass was placed on my face, and removed to dry, forming a hard mask. Each treatment, my skull was tightened to the table while wearing the hardened mask to keep my head from moving during radiation.

Paul and we were concerned there may be other unseen plasmacytomas. Tests showed no others, but my abnormal protein continued to rise. He wanted me to add Velcade to the maintenance myeloma drug I was already taking. I questioned whether, instead, my dose of maintenance drug could be increased to see if that reduced the abnormal protein. He disagreed and wanted to add Velcade. My goal was to save Velcade in case the myeloma got out of control. We knew it worked well earlier, and there were no other new myeloma drugs at that time. I was comfortable with my risk in part since only one plasmacytoma developed while I was taking the maintenance drug.

We seemed to be at an impasse, when my Dana clinical trial nurse and friend, Debby spoke up and said she wanted to talk with me separately. She offered a compromise, since she worked with both of us, "Jim, you will not convince Paul with your myeloma judgment; he is the myeloma expert. Try letting Paul know you would be more comfortable keeping Velcade in reserve for when it may be needed more."

When I explained my feelings to Paul, he said that while he did not recommend my way, he would go along with me, providing CT and PET scans revealed no other plasmacytomas, and I would agree to add Velcade if the abnormal protein did not decline after a month of increased higher dose of the current drug I was taking when the plasmacytoma appeared. I agreed.

The scans showed no other plasmacytomas, and I increased my maintenance drug. When I called Paul the next month to report the abnormal protein declined, I was unsure of how he would respond. He put me at ease by saying, "Good call, Jim."

To me, this was another example of teamwork with our medical team and how fortunate we are to have Paul R and Debby D, among others.

Medical research, top-flight medical teams, good fortune, great support, and hard work enabled me to survive.

POHR Memories

I value many memories from annually riding a bike 4 days across Ohio's scenic bike trails and country roads each year. Riding part of the route with Jim, Bob and other family created great moments we may not have shared without the POHR. I was ready to give up from exhaustion day 3 of the first ride. Jim was riding with me up a long hill several miles from Antioch College where we were staying that night. We stopped and talked about the cold beer and celebrating at the upcoming night's campus, got back on our bikes, and Jim led the way to the day's finish, where riders were waiting to greet us.

The same year, another rider, Tom Brennan, dropped back from the pack of riders to ride and talk with me at the slower pace I cycle. After we exchanged our background stories on why we were riding to help cancer patients, Tom said he had an elderly relative who was recently diagnosed with a rare blood cancer and was struggling. Tom asked me to meet his relative, Delmar Littleton, at our upcoming lunch stop in Danville, a small Ohio farming community.

When I met Delmar and his wife Helen, I asked how he was doing, and he said, "I am not doing well with the medication my local doctor prescribed, and I am sad hearing from my doctor that no one has survived my type of cancer for more than 3 years."

I asked the name of his blood cancer and the drug he was taking, and Delmar said, "I have multiple myeloma", and he named the drug he was struggling with.

I was shocked at the coincidence, and replied that I also have myeloma, have lived 15 years, and am cycling 4 days across Ohio. The sudden change in their expressions was dramatic. Helen's sadness turned into a big smile—a sight that lives in my memory. I added that I had taken the same drug without problems and suggested that his doctor contact my doctor to discuss the dose Delmar was receiving. The following year, Delmar told me his medication was adjusted and he was doing well. It was POHR karma in action.

Delmar returned to that lunch stop for about five years, and we became close. He was like another father figure to me. He passed away from a heart condition. Kathleen and I drove over a hundred miles to attend Delmar's funeral. We were emotional when we saw that among the memorial pictures on display was the POHR shirt Kathleen had given him years earlier. We are still in contact with his relative Tom. The Danville POHR lunch stop bears Delmar's name.

POHR's initial year memories include Bob's wife, Stacey, training and riding part of the route with me. We rode into a sudden thunderstorm, with lightning and thunder, and took cover on a farmer's porch until the storm cleared. Stacey and I continue to talk about that unwanted excitement.

Kathleen was only able to get two ACS staffers assigned to the first POHR. She had few volunteers outside of northeast Ohio. It's amazing that Kathleen and her tiny crew could lead all 50 of us riders safely over 4 days. Later, she told me, behind the scenes, it was a fire drill, finishing one water stop, loading unused food and drink in the car and racing to set up for the next water stop.

This challenge is compounded by our riders arriving at stops, meals and our dorms at different times, because riders' paces vary. Looking back, it seems impossible that it went so smoothly from a rider's perspective She knew it was vital to have riders pleased with their POHR experience, to spread the word.

When I was diagnosed and began chemo treatments, my nurse was a new UH nurse, Anne Kolenic. She knew about the upcoming initial POHR and that volunteers were needed. Anne quietly organized nurse colleagues and surprised me at our day 1 lunch stop not too far from UH, where she became a leader and earned a PhD.

Another memory of that first POHR is arriving at our day 4 finish, the ACS Cincinnati Hope Lodge. The previous day, some of our faster riders asked Kathleen if it would be OK if they waited for us slow riders so we could all ride into the finish together. This was a turning point for the POHR. Our expert cyclists understood the POHR was not about cycling, it was about helping people with cancer. It brought tears to Kathleen's eyes to see her idea become a reality.

Men in Scottish kilts were playing bagpipes for us in front of the Hope Lodge. Jim was riding next to me, with his camera recording. Patient and caregiver residents at the Hope Lodge were waving their welcome.

Other UH nurses who treated me, including Lee Shetina, Leslie Craig and Linda Baer volunteered at future years lunch stops. Linda became a physician assistant and continues to help manage my case and provide her valuable judgment.

Kathleen invited my current UH doctor, Marcos DeLima, to a POHR kick off dinner in Cleveland. Marcos not only helped with my last transplant, but he also took over my myeloma and related issues. Marcos and Linda are more than outstanding medical professionals, they are friends who we rely upon.

Would there be a POHR had I not gotten diagnosed with myeloma? Maybe, but her care giving for me likely played a part in her idea.

When asked if Kathleen founded POHR to help her husband, I reply, "Kathleen founded and lead the POHR to help all cancer patients, not just me."

Several other ACS multi-day bike rides resulted from the successful POHR and are annual events in other states. I could not be prouder of her leadership and determination.

Lastly, Stacey and Bob gave me a gift years ago with a picture of me, alone, struggling as I cycled up one of the country hills in POHR. Teddy Roosevelt's famous quote was on the picture.

It says not to criticize a person who gives his all, whether successful or not. Give credit to the person in the struggle, or Arena.

I am humbled and honored Stacey and Bob suggested this as part of my book title.

Life is Good

Bob, Stacey and their daughter, Jillian, moved from Chicago to a house nearby us.

Bob enrolled at Case Western Reserve University in Cleveland to earn an MBA. We were happy to have more time with all three of them without the need to travel.

I enjoyed helping Bob with a small part of his kitchen remodeling. We watched Jillian play soccer, basketball, and softball. I enjoyed tossing the ball with her in the backyard. We enjoyed trips to Chicago to visit Jim, Emilee, and their growing family, as our grandsons, Dayton and then Wade arrived. Dayton and Wade did POHR fundraising from their lemonade stand.

Kathleen and I continued to travel the country sharing our survival story with ACS audiences and with myeloma support groups as part of myeloma programs we were invited to join. We would arrange to take a few days' vacation on some trips to explore areas we had never seen. When I reached age 60 after 39 years with the firm, I was required to retire from our EY partnership, and vacation days were no longer a constraint. We saw parts of the country for the first time, including the Grand Canyon and the Naval Base in San Diego.

MDS (Myelodysplastic Syndrome)

My blood counts began to worsen. Thankfully, abnormal protein was not increasing, suggesting the myeloma was stable and likely not the cause. A bone marrow biopsy was done, confirming myeloma was stable, but my bone marrow was not producing normal blood counts, requiring close monitoring.

Counts continued to decline, and another biopsy showed that MDS (myelodysplasia syndrome) had developed causing the low blood counts. I recall the UH transplant doctor explained that my MDS will almost assuredly lead to leukemia, and he recommended the MDS be immediately treated as if it were leukemia.

I told him we needed time to consider his recommendation. After some research and thinking, we decided to seek a second opinion from another hospital, since there seemed to be some question as to whether the MDS would lead to leukemia. I contacted Paul R at Dana and asked him to suggest a colleague who has experience in this area. He recommended Dr. Daniel DeAngelo who led their adult leukemia group as well as Dr. Joseph Antin in their stem cell transplant unit.

I wanted to avoid an unnecessary bone marrow biopsy, but Dana doctors needed to review my marrow slides. I asked that my UH biopsy slides be sent to Dana for Dan D. and Joe A. to review in advance of our appointments. The UH transplant doctor, I recall did not seem thrilled that we decided not to immediately proceed to treat the MDS as leukemia. I think he believed I was making a mistake.

I reviewed my summary of monthly blood counts and saw that the counts were only declining slowly, not rapidly. I felt the time for a second opinion was worthwhile.

Our meetings were insightful. Paul R helped by providing these doctors with our history and background. Joe A. believed the type of leukemia that MDS may lead to can be successfully treated. Dan D. focused on my key question: "Do you agree with the UH transplant doctor's opinion my MDS would almost certainly lead to leukemia, and that treatment should begin now?"

After Dan D. paused, he indicated he did not agree. In his opinion the MDS may or may not lead to leukemia. He suggested continued close monitoring of my blood counts and doing another bone marrow biopsy if the white counts or platelets show significant decline. We decided to follow this "watch and wait" type of approach. It later proved to be a key decision.

Year from Hell

2012 hit our family like a tornado. I started my POHR bike training early due to a warm spring. To be cautious, I use quiet streets close to our house for my training route. Starting one day's ride, I fainted while cycling at my normal moderate pace. I woke up in a hospital's critical care unit, and Kathleen was at my side to explain what happened.

A police officer had knocked on our front door and told her I had a bike accident, and an ambulance was on the way. When she asked where it happened, he pointed to a curve in the street several houses from ours. A neighbor saw me crash, helmet first to the ground and called the police. My helmet likely saved my life. It was badly cracked, but it did its job.

They diagnosed a brain hematoma and a fractured collar bone. The impact to my head was causing the loss of feeling or movement to one leg. After a couple of days in that hospital, I was able to feel and move my leg. My arm was put in a sling, making it difficult to use crutches to walk. Heart and brain specialists ran tests and found nothing else wrong. An ambulance was ordered to take me to their physical therapy unit for admission to rehabilitate my leg.

Kathleen stepped in and said, "I will take Jim in our car to UH's physical therapy unit. UH knows Jim's history very well and we need to go there."

I spent over a week rehabilitating my leg before I was discharged, able to walk out without crutches. I was referred to a UH neurologist to diagnose why I fainted, and why occasional lightheadedness was occurring. The UH neurologist agreed with the neurologist at the hospital who earlier examined me after my accident. Neither could find the cause. They gave the disappointing news that I would have to live with occasional lightheadedness.

Things seemed tough but I was very lucky it wasn't worse. Shortly thereafter, things went from bad to worse. Our teenage granddaughter, Jillian, died by suicide. Jillian had been dealing with a lot problems that many teenage girls face and we thought she was overcoming her challenges; however, it took a turn. We were all devastated, certainly no more so than her parents, Stacey and Bob, who had done everything they could to ensure that Jillian had the best therapists and opportunities. To say it was tragic feels like an understatement. We came together as a family to support one another through it, but one never gets over such loss, you learn to live with it.

I was back to bike training, and being especially careful, stopping when I felt the slightest bit of fatigue. One weekend, Kathleen dropped me off to bike several miles on a scenic bike path in the Cuyahoga Valley National Park, not too far from our house. I stopped a few times when I felt fatigue, got back on and cycled more. We met at a casual outdoor restaurant near the bike path. In the middle of dinner, I fainted, my face landing on my sandwich and fries.

Kathleen helped me sit upright, and the restaurant called an ambulance which took me to the nearest emergency room. The emergency medical staff observed me as I began to feel normal. They wanted to admit me for further tests, but I declined, and we went home, with my promise to call our family doctor, Kevin Geraci, on Monday.

When I told Kevin about both fainting episodes, occasional lightheadedness, and heart and brain specialists concluding there was nothing they could do, he said, "Jim come into the office, we'll get to the bottom of this."

Kevin G arranged for me to see a cardiologist in his UH hospital unit, even though another cardiologist had tested my heart while hospitalized for the bike crash. Kevin's friend explained that my heart needed to be tested not while lying in a hospital bed as was done after the bike crash, but when I was going through my normal daily activities. He put several sensors on my chest wired to a monitoring device. I wore the harness for two days and recorded what I was doing when I felt faint and was told to stay off the bike.

When Kevin's cardiologist colleague reviewed the results, he said, "Jim, you need a pacemaker, your heart is not pumping enough blood to your brain when you exert yourself. A pacemaker will fix this."

He was right, immediately after the UH surgeon, Ivan Cakulev, put in a pacemaker, I was back to normal.

As I was entering surgery, I jokingly asked Ivan if he could set the pacemaker to make me feel twenty years younger. Kathleen replied first and said, "Not unless I have a remote control."

We have not lost our sense of humor. It helps us.

I completed my training and was feeling safe about riding in the annual event. My family encouraged me to take a year off, but something made me ride again. My UH medical team gave me a drug to increase my red blood count to a normal level, making it easier to ride.

As I had previously done, I completed all four days of the POHR without an accident. Jim, Bob and Stacey also rode that year.

Two months after the POHR, my outstanding UH infusion room nurse, Lee Shetina, asked me to stop in for labs before our next trip. She felt I looked a little pale. When she came back with the blood results, the look on Lee's face said it all. Something was very wrong.

She said, "Jim, your platelets have drastically dropped to such a dangerously low reading that it could cause bleeding while flying at high altitude. You need to cancel today's trip and get a bone marrow biopsy now to see what's going on."

I reminded Lee I've had 38 bone marrow biopsies and asked if she was sure I had to have another bone marrow biopsy.

"Yes, we're very sure, Jim" she said.

The UH transplant doctor called two days later and said, "Bad news, Jim, your MDS led to leukemia (the AML variety). Worse than that, yours is treatment-related leukemia, which means the only way you can survive is to get another allo transplant, if we can reduce the leukemia level and then find a match for you."

I reminded him my sister matches me, and he said, "Your bone marrow thinks you are your sister, and her stem cells will not work. We need to search the national bone marrow data base to see if an unrelated matching donor exists. But we are ahead of ourselves; your bone marrow is compromised from three previous transplants; you are 64; this would be very difficult. You may want to discuss this with Kathleen and let me know what you decide."

I said she was listening, and I will see you tomorrow to begin. That was our wedding anniversary, and we went out and celebrated as best we could. We were grateful for all our prior anniversaries and being able to be together.

I am grateful the UH transplant doctor gave me the option to try to survive leukemia.

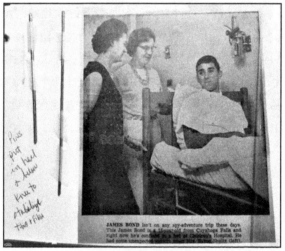

Baseball injury ended one dream, but good things resulted later

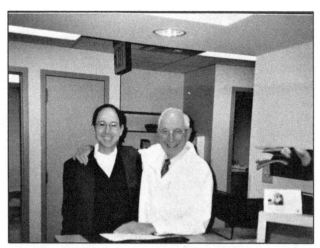

Bob Kellermeyer got us started, with his valuable
strategies, skill and compassion

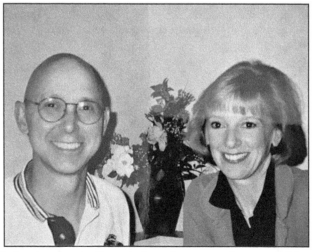

Remission is a happy time, but we knew myeloma would return

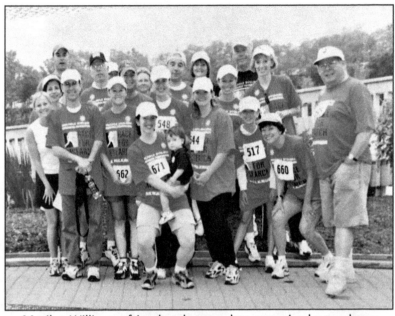

Marilyn Willis, my friend and co-worker, organized a myeloma
fundraiser with friends & family

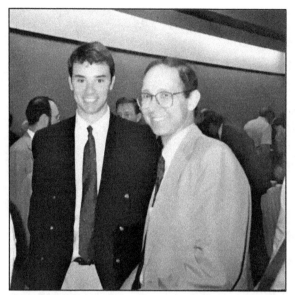

Surprising Jim at his college graduation. Thanks,
University Hospitals of Cleveland

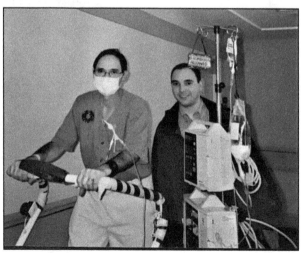

Nurses put treadmill by my room; Bob visited transplant floor

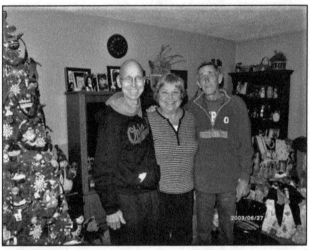

With sister, Becki, and brother-in-law, Dan Kramer, a best friend

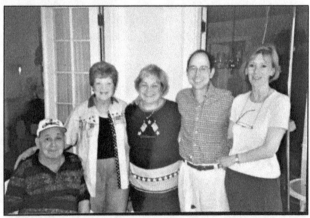

Last time with my Dad. Pat and Becki visited before
we relocated to Boston

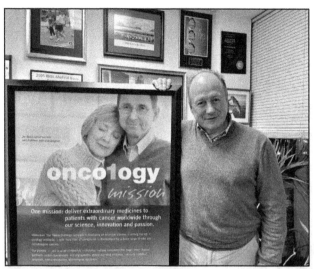

Paul Richardson led the Dana Farber clinical trial team that saved my life and helped get Velcade approved in record time.

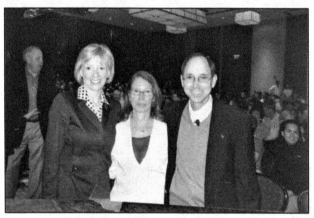

Us with Velcade Clinical Nurse, Debby Doss, RN at Millennium Pharma celebration

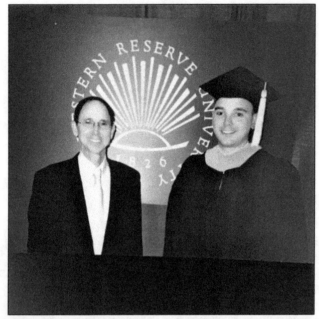

Bob earned an MBA from Case Western Reserve University

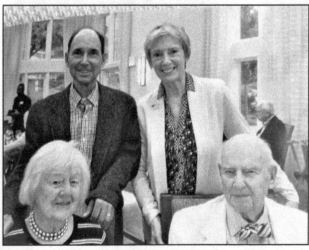

Our last visit with Sandy and Joan Cunningham. We miss Sandy.

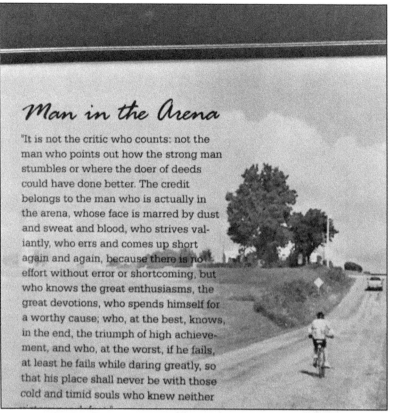

Man in the Arena

"It is not the critic who counts: not the man who points out how the strong man stumbles or where the doer of deeds could have done better. The credit belongs to the man who is actually in the arena, whose face is marred by dust and sweat and blood, who strives valiantly, who errs and comes up short again and again, because there is no effort without error or shortcoming, but who knows the great enthusiasms, the great devotions, who spends himself for a worthy cause; who, at the best, knows, in the end, the triumph of high achievement, and who, at the worst, if he fails, at least he fails while daring greatly, so that his place shall never be with those cold and timid souls who knew neither

Stacey and Bob gave me this POHR pic with "Man in the Arena" quote and suggested using Teddy Roosevelt's quote in naming this book.

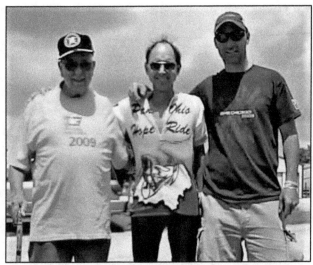

Delmar Littleton, Jim and me at Danville, OH
lunch stop, named for Delmar

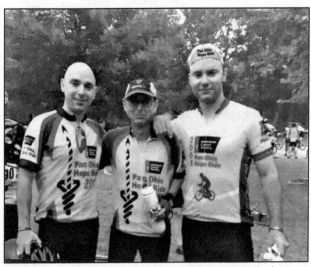

Bob, me and Jim at water stop on our POHR 100 mile 'century' day.

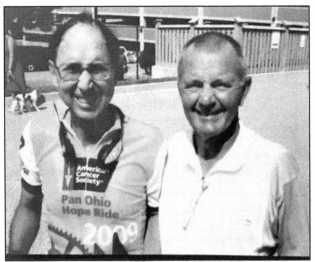

Dennis Hoffer, good friend and POHR co-founder, ensures Ohio bike routes are the safest and scenic.

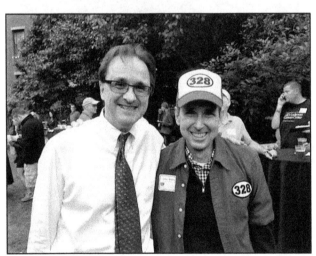

Marcos deLima at our POHR kick off dinner before Day 1 start the next morning. Marcos, Linda Baer, Lee Shetina and their UH Seidman Cancer Center team got me through difficult situations, with world-class skill and compassion.

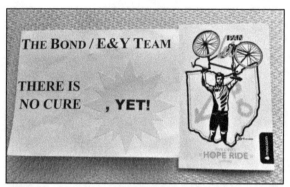

Marilyn Willis, my friend and coworker, made "yet" stickers and Jim made POHR cards to advocate for curing cancer.

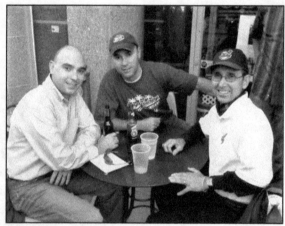

Bob and Jim with me before an Indians playoff game in Cleveland.

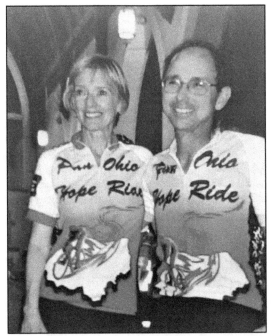

Us celebrating the first ACS Pan Ohio Hope Ride,
at the finish in Cincinnati

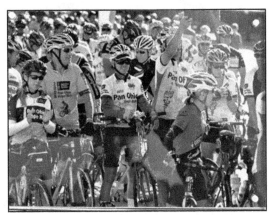

Many riders joined us at Kathleen's POHR. Each year was like a
family reunion. Some riders say the POHR impacted their lives.

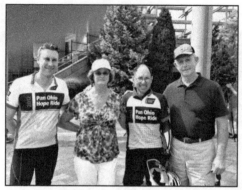

My friend Craig Brooks with Tom Brennan and his wife Mary Anne. Tom rode with me in first POHR, and years later, he emotionally greeted us near his home.

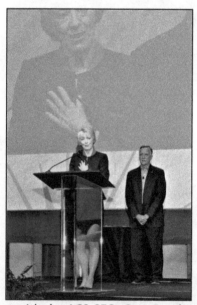

In 2017 Kathleen with the ACS CEO, Gary Reedy, receiving ACS's highest national volunteer leader award in Atlanta. Jim flew in, and Kathleen's sister Mary Ann and daughter, Sammy, drove all night to surprise her.

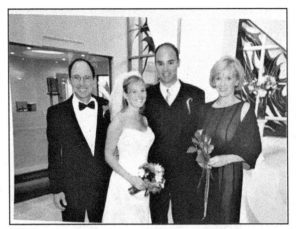

In 2002, I was given time off from my Velcade trial
to enjoy Emilee's & Jim's wedding.

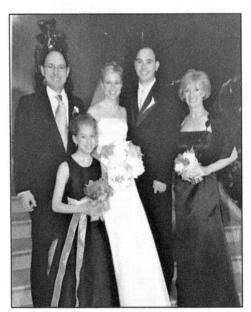

Proud parents and grandparents with Stacey, Jillian
and Bob at their 2004 wedding.

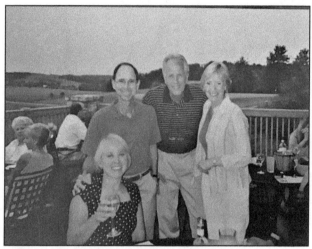

My sister, Denyse and husband, Charlie Patterson
at dinner, near Granville, OH

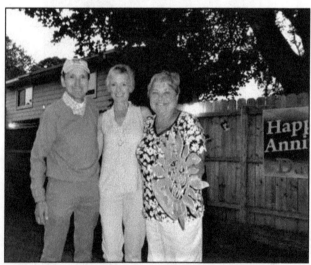

Celebrating my sister, Becki's and Dan Kramer's 50th wedding
anniversary at their daughter Amy's and Mardy's home in Stow, OH

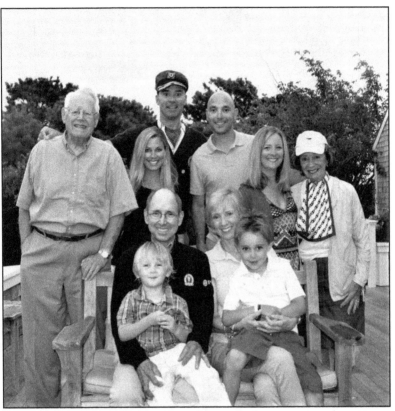

With Kathleen's parents, Bob and Mae, and our gang on vacation.

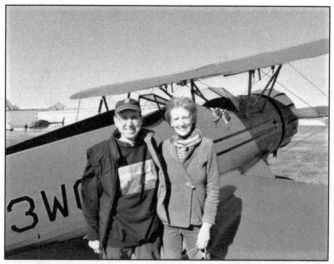

Getting ready for an open-cockpit biplane ride in Arizona on vacation.

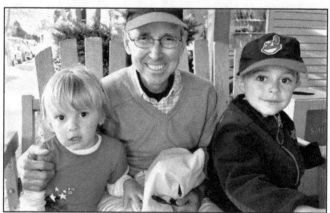

Wade, Dayton and me in western Michigan.

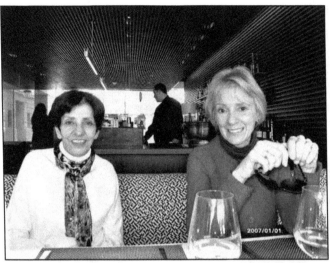

Sunday breakfast at Yours Truly, solving world problems.

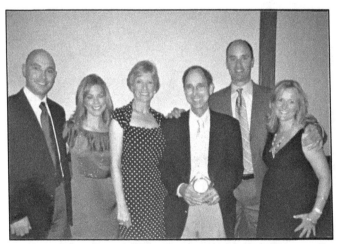

Us celebrating my EY retirement with Bob, Stacey,
Jim and Emilee Bond

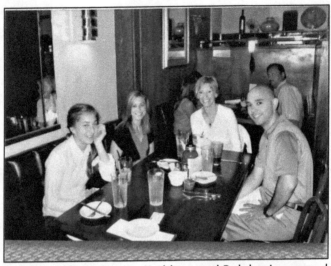

Granddaughter Jillian, Stacey, Kathleen and Bob having a good time.

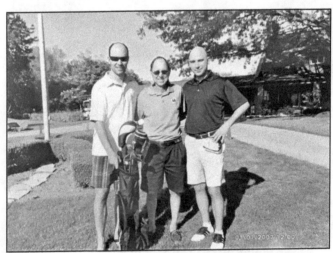

Jim, Bob and I after another great time golfing
together in Shaker Heights

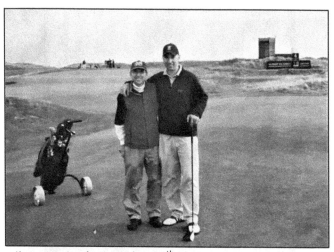

Jim surprised me with a 60th birthday trip to Scotland,
and legendary courses.

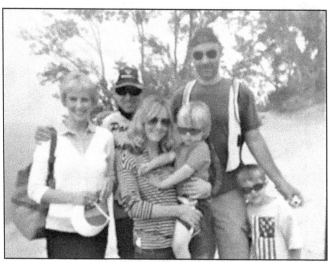

We had lots of fun with Emilee, Jim, Dayton and Wade
on a western MI vacation

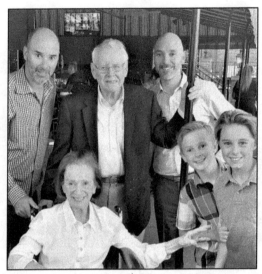

We surprised Kathleen on her 70th birthday. Above are her parents, our sons and grandsons and our extended families traveled to Shaker Heights to celebrate.

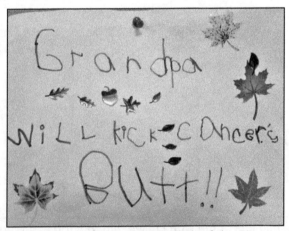

Grandson Dayton's optimism made each of the 75 consecutive hospital days brighter, as did his brother Wade's artwork on my wall.

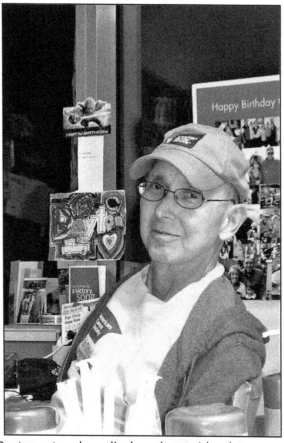

More Dayton artwork on display, along with other memories to cheer me. Note the striped bass Jim caught in the surf with me and the family enjoyed eating.

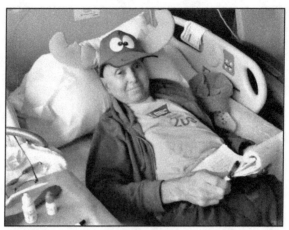

Halloween during transplant number 4; drugs have me lying down with my medical pad and pen.

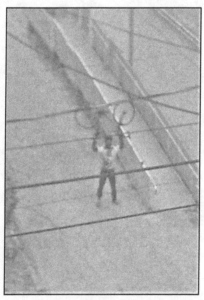

Jim called and said, "Dad, look out your transplant window." He uplifted my spirit during transplant number 4. Jim flew from Chicago and biked from our house to surprise me.

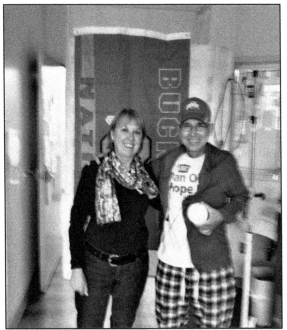

My sister, Denyse, and Charlie visited during leukemia transplant, bringing Buckeye Karma.

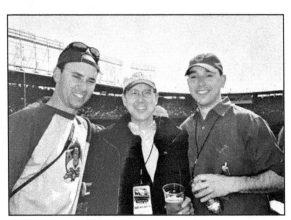

Jim and me at Bob's bachelor party overlooking Wrigley Field.

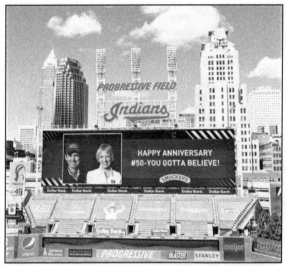

The Indians announcing our 50th during a game.
Kathleen really surprised me.

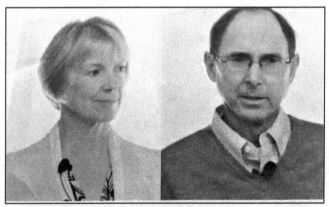

Dallas 2011 Support group talk, looking serious.

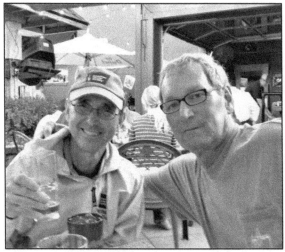

Best man at our wedding, Roy Burnett, my good friend and fishing buddy. Now two old guys remembering good old days and loving it.

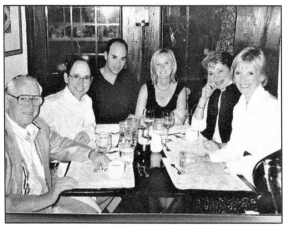

Kathleen's parents, Jim, and Emilee enjoying time with each other.

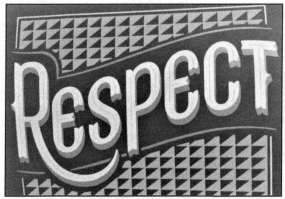

Patient acronym I developed, along with other acronyms in the book

Leukemia

Each of my previous three transplants presented differing degrees of difficulty, which is why having UH's top-notch transplant medical team is so fortunate. This fourth transplant was the most difficult, by far.

I was admitted for what turned out to be 75 consecutive days. Being in UH's new Seidman Cancer Center helped. The transplant had rooms with large windows, and the floor had an exercise room with a treadmill. Kathleen was with me every day, and visits with our sons, daughters-in-law, and other family and friends helped a lot. Son, Jim, generously made frequent surprise visits from Chicago. One day, Emilee flew over and back from Chicago to visit and she continually sent notes from the kids. Our grandsons, Dayton and Wade, sent lots of artwork to cheer me, which I proudly hung on my door.

One of Dayton's posters said, "Grandpa is going to kick cancer's butt."

The on-duty transplant doctors and nurses were not as optimistic. I quickly noticed they were seemingly trying to lower my expectations, and I kept encouraging them we could do this.

I developed a fungal infection that the UH team correctly treated like one of the worst types, aspergillus, for my safety reasons. I did the required tests before starting the transplant process.

I began receiving heavy chemotherapy doses for the long transplant process.

In one 3-day period, I hallucinated for the first and only time in my life. Things appeared to me that were not actually there. The imaginary things were still present when I closed my eyes, and nothing was good about the images. These were my worst days and nights in dealing with cancer or transplants.

Kathleen's comfort got me through by assuring me it would pass in a few days. I trust her. The UH veteran pharmacist and experienced transplant doctors could not understand the cause. Kathleen later offered a cause no one had considered: the brain hematoma from my earlier bike crash and chemo drugs could have triggered the hallucinations. No one had a better explanation.

My sister, Becki played another critical part when I needed platelets as the ones from the normal source were failing to stay with me very long. My bone marrow was not yet producing my own blood cells, and it was getting tense. Since we know her stem cells matched mine, she donated her platelets. This was again hard for Becki because of her fear of blood and needles in her arm, but she donated despite her fear. Her platelets stayed in me the normal amount of time, and the tension eased.

Again, I forced myself to sit, stand or walk depending on how much strength I could muster that day. At some point, Dr. Marcos deLima (Marcos) a new member of the transplant team helped care for me. He is like a few of my oncology doctors. I think he sees the half full part of the glass, not the half empty part. Yet, he does not hold back information. Bob K, Paul R and Kevin G share this outlook, which means a lot to me.

On a Sunday night, after Kathleen was back home from her daily visit, and the long hospital confinement was getting old, my phone rang, and I heard, "Paul Richardson here. I just talked to Kathleen, and I want to repeat what I told her. We have had other myeloma patients who developed leukemia. They were able to make it through the difficult transplant, and you will do the same."

Paul's words meant a lot to both of us and helped a lot.

As another bone marrow biopsy confirmed, heavy chemo doses drove down the leukemia level to permit another allo transplant, and a matching donor was found on the national and international bone marrow data base! This was the big news we were praying for.

I was very happy and asked, "When can I receive the unrelated donor's stem cells?"

The reply was devastating.

I recall the transplant doctor saying, "The UH transplant doctors approval board does not believe you are a good risk to survive another allo transplant. All members must approve it, and more than one is voting against you."

I said that since I would die if I did not get the allo transplant, why not give it a try? The response was that they knew that was true, but they could not be the ones who took my life. I tried other ways to convince them, but none seemed to help.

The UH transplant doctor came a day later and I recall the UH transplant doctor saying, "Jim, when I did as you asked and told the skeptical transplant doctors you rode your bike 328 miles in 4 days less than two months ago, they changed their minds. They realized you must be strong enough both physically and mentally to get through it. We now have all doctors voting yes on the transplant."

We again witnessed how suddenly things can change in dealing with a deadly blood cancer. It felt like we were on an emotional roller coaster.

I received the donor's stem cells on Halloween. Another bone marrow biopsy indicated I was in remission for the leukemia, and myeloma remained in remission. I was discharged before Christmas and we were grateful 2012 was ending. I remain in remission today.

I am very grateful for what the UH transplant doctor and his team did for me to get me through four transplants.

At times this UH transplant doctor and I had different views, which added tension. We seemed to overcome our differences, in part due to our common ground, baseball.

Had I decided not to ride in the 2012 POHR, this transplant would not have happened. This is true because cycling those four days changed the minds of skeptical doctors to vote yes. In my view, the ACS saved my life again. First, by funding scientists whose fundamental research opened the door to the development of Velcade, and now by supporting Kathleen's idea to launch the POHR years ago. I am very grateful to the ACS.

Marcos also told me and others I made it through this transplant because I made myself get out of bed, even on days when he knew I felt poorly.

Bone Marrow Registry

Two years later I learned my donor was a young woman living in Germany who had registered on the bone marrow data base. I could not thank her enough for saving my life. Her being German may also explain why since this transplant, I have had an urge to go to Octoberfest.

We encourage people age 18 to 44 to consider registering on the donor data base. Searching "Be the Match" has simple, no cost instructions. From their kit, rubbing a Q-tip on the inside of your mouth and returning it is all that is needed. Once registered, a potential donor can always change their mind, if they become a match. I am grateful for the National Bone Marrow Registry and its lifesaving work.

A friend and employee of Takeda Oncology, Sabina McCafferty, led a campaign for her colleagues to register. She also touched me by visiting me in the hospital.

Our Approach

As Kathleen puts it: we've tried to do what was necessary, then try to do what's possible, and when we look back, we feel like we've accomplished what seemed impossible when cancer entered our lives.

The most important thing I learned about allo transplants is that having a transplant hospital with experienced transplant doctors and staff is critical. Expert allo medical knowledge and experience are needed to judge the intensity of the allo transplant. One size does not fit all. I am grateful my transplants were done by what I consider top-notch transplant doctors and staff and UH's Seidman Cancer Center.

There are key approaches we've used throughout. Trying to learn as much as we could and to keep up with new developments is one. Myeloma was overwhelming at the beginning and trying to digest everything at once was not possible. Over time we saw myeloma as a marathon, not a sprint. At times, we had to exert all our energy to keep going, but we reminded ourselves there would be more normal times ahead. Taking one challenge at a time worked best. We continue to learn from experiences of other patients and caregivers as well as our medical teams.

To keep more options open, I try to stay on the current myeloma drug until it is no longer effective for me, saving unused ones for later when they may be needed.

We try not to look back once we've made a decision.

We try to become equal partners with my doctors, nurses, and in a few cases, medical technicians. It would be foolish to try to be the boss of what we view as a team, with each member bringing its own knowledge and skill. Myeloma doctors know much more about cancer and treatments, and after many years, we know more about our case history and risk tolerance. Combining these has worked for us. Other patients may prefer a different approach, and I agree we should each do what feels right. Each case is unique since each of our bodies differ. We've learned to avoid internet material that is more personal opinion and unsubstantiated than sound, medical findings.

As earlier mentioned, daily exercise is a cornerstone of my patient and Kathleen's caregiver approach. Fatigue, medications, and frustration can make this hard for me. Kathleen believes taking care of herself cannot be overlooked because when I am struggling, she is a more effective caregiver when she feels healthy. She takes time for her exercise, whatever form it takes.

After coming home from my first transplant, I had permission to walk outside. I started by setting a modest goal of walking to the end of our block and back. I gradually challenged myself to keep going farther from our house, eventually feeling stronger. When I have a myeloma setback, I've learned to accept being able to do less exercise. The phrases "Sit, Stand, and Walk" and "On my Feet not my Seat" describe my goals that change with the circumstances.

After a couple years, Kathleen and I agreed on what we call our "Eight PM Rule". At 8 PM we are done talking about cancer—with each other or someone else. Whatever decision or new thought we may have will have to wait until tomorrow. We've found doing this helps us have a little more time to relax before we go to bed. We try to follow this rule, whether I'm hospitalized or not. Kathleen likes to point out this originally was a 9 PM rule, but we're older now. She also adds, "If it ever becomes a 7 PM rule, we're not telling anyone."

We believe in clinical trials and second opinions when appropriate for us. We have had several second opinions from other cancer centers that focus on myeloma patients.

I've been in six clinical trials—3 for experimental drugs and 3 transplants which had at least one clinical trial element. I would only enter a clinical trial if I thought it was my best option. My thinking is that if the procedure or experimental drug is not effective, other patients may benefit from clinical trial findings. Our experience is that my care was at least as good, or better, in each clinical trial, than when treated outside a trial.

We have heard and read objections that prevent some patients from entering a clinical trial. Everyone should do what they are comfortable doing. Our experiences have been positive. For example, when one experimental drug was not effective for me, the doctor quickly took me off that trial and offered another option. I have never felt like my health was secondary to the clinical trial.

We have gotten several second opinions, and each has added to our knowledge and helped us make decisions that we were more comfortable making. If a doctor may feel badly about our getting a second opinion, I put my life before their feelings. We are fortunate that virtually all my doctors understood my seeking a second opinion. I believe most doctors are like mine, placing their patient's health first. I know a couple other patients who were not so fortunate when their local doctor warned the patient if he went to a major myeloma center for a second opinion, the local doctor would stop seeing him.

That friend and patient contacted me and asked what I would do, and I said, "I would leave that local doctor and ask the second opinion doctor to recommend another local doctor close to my home."

My friend did this and has monthly visits with his new local doctor for more routine procedures, saving him monthly long-distance trips. He periodically visits the myeloma center. Many other patients, including me, find this approach works well. A few rare times one of my local doctors became frustrated, feeling like he was a second-class citizen to the out-of-town myeloma specialist. I believe it is my role to help work out an acceptable compromise.

Another key approach is being compliant with what our doctor and we agree to do. There are times when the preference of my doctor differs from mine, but once an agreement is reached, I do my best to comply. Kathleen is vital to my complying with my medication timing and doses. She ensures prescriptions are filled and fills a container of each day's morning and afternoon pills. I am very grateful to have such a hard-working caregiver.

Caregivers ask Kathleen how she copes with the stress, especially when I am taking high doses of a steroid. She believes it helps to sometimes just let all her emotions out. She adds that a spouse on steroids is, "Why rooms have doors on them."

Our sons had a hat made for me saying "Captain Chaos" to put some humor in our situation.

After the Velcade clinical trial, my long-time doctor, Bob K, wrote a congratulatory letter, and said, "I think the other reason you are alive is that you are the most compliant cancer patient I have had in my long career."

I thanked Bob K and said I could not imagine a patient not complying when they were dealing with something as serious as cancer. He said unfortunately there are patients who are not good at complying. When Bob K started treating me, he said my myeloma impairs my kidneys when monoclonal protein is high. He recommended that I drink plenty of fluids daily to help my kidney impairment. I follow that advice and try to always stay hydrated.

We have learned the importance of continuing to make long-term plans, despite uncertainties of cancer. Plans can be changed if necessary and looking forward to planned vacations or family gatherings helps us. A newly diagnosed friend met with us to discuss approaches we take. A few years later, this friend called to thank me for our advice.

I was not sure what he was referring to until he said, "We said that we had hoped to someday visit Italy, and we were sad that myeloma would prevent this dream from happening. You told us to make our plans anyway. I want you to know we just returned from Italy."

Not all Good News

Myeloma, leukemia, and treatments have had adverse effects. I am about three inches shorter, and twenty pounds lighter than at diagnosis. My spine is somewhat twisted and curved. I saw one old friend who had not seen me in many years, and he was visibly shocked I was smaller.

My one shoulder's joint was destroyed, causing limited range of motion with that arm, but no ongoing pain. That arm is about an inch shorter that the other. I continue to golf with both hands on the clubs, but the one arm is only going along for the ride, not adding anything. My golf game was never good. I golf to be outdoors and walk with enjoyable people.

After the unrelated donor transplant, my eyesight was so bad I had to stop driving, and my constantly irritated eyes stung, and I needed to squint. My family and friends thought I always looked angry. Ocular Graft vs Host disease (GVHD) was the cause. My doctors explained that while my donor's stem cells matched mine, her cells also adversely reacted to other body parts. I understand a little GVHD is a good thing—it confirms that her stem cells continue to fight my cancers, but excessive GVHD creates difficulties, such as my eye problems.

My local eye doctors could not find a solution to return my eyesight and help my eye irritation, despite a frustrating year of trying different eye drops and a second doctor. When I asked Marcos if he had any ideas, he recommended a colleague of his at a well-known Houston cancer center where he previously practiced. While I was trying to schedule an appointment, Kathleen did research which showed that Houston doctor trained in Boston at Massachusetts Eye and Ear Infirmary (MEEI). Since we visited Dana in Boston twice a year for myeloma checkups, we instead scheduled an appointment with their doctor who had trained Marcos's recommendation.

The MEEI doctor tried a couple new eye drops with slight success for about a year, and then said, "Since drops are not helping, a specialty provider called BostonSight may be able to help."

BostonSight doctor, Alan Kwok, and staff examined my eyes. He asked how irritated my eyes felt, and I rated the pain as 6 on a scale of 10 being the worst. He then took out an oversized hard contact lens, filled it with liquid, pulled open my eye lids and inserted the huge lens in one eye. It was done so quickly, I thought he may have dropped the lens. I opened my eyes, and all my irritation in that eye was instantly gone, and my eyesight in that eye returned to normal.

Kathleen was amazed my one eye was now wide open and the look on my face immediately went from a frown to a smile. I said, "Doctor, I need to change my earlier answer; my pain level was a 9 or 10—not the six that I earlier reported."

I lived with my eye irritation so long, I had become used to it and it was affecting not only my eyes, but my life. Alan Kwok used their proprietary procedures and BostonSight made the huge contact lenses, using laser technology to exactly fit my eyes within a couple of days. Alan Kwok explained these unique lenses were called PROSE devices, which are similar to scleral lenses, except they are made specifically for the exact size and shape of each of my eyes and they rest on the white part of my eyes.

We checked in to a nearby hotel for the scheduled 2 weeks training I would need to learn to insert and remove the devices daily. We were very fortunate our training technician, Heidi Wolf, was top-notch and compassionate. I had only worn eyeglasses, never contacts. Removing and inserting the lenses required both hands—one to hold the eyelids far apart with my fingers, and the other hand to hold a small rubber device to suction each lens on and off my eye. Insertion was done by balancing a lens on another rubber device, like a golf ball on a tee. I filled the lens with a liquid before each insertion. The limited range of one arm gave me trouble learning the technique.

After two weeks training ended, and I was in my third week, I had frustrated myself and the staff. I was struggling to master the technique. Alan Kwok asked me if I wanted to quit trying. But Heidi told me, "Jim, I do not want to hear you complain about your bad shoulder. I helped another patient with only one arm learn to do this."

With renewed motivation from Heidi, I finally learned well enough to go home with PROSE devices in my eyes. They showed Kathleen how to step in if I needed help inserting or removing the devices. My eyesight and life returned to normal. I am grateful to Heidi for not giving up on me. We continue to have annual checkups at BostonSight.

My stomach, skin and mouth also are affected by GVHD, but not nearly to the extent my eyes are, and new GVHD medication became available in the last couple of years that helps relieve my symptoms.

I earlier mentioned I am at high risk for skin cancer said to be due to transplant effects on my immune system. My UH dermatologists explained just one transplant can cause this. I see the dermatologist every 3 or 4 months, and they almost always find skin cancer spots, but never melanoma, which took my youngest sister, Janell's, life when she was only 40.

My one hip required replacing, said to be due to long-term effects of steroids required for certain myeloma treatments, as previously mentioned. I am now cautious about agreeing to add a steroid to a treatment protocol since my hip experience.

After my first three transplants, I developed shingles. My cases were fairly mild. My thyroid stopped working, which may or may not be a cancer side effect. Daily medication handles my thyroid problem.

It was difficult to diagnose. Kathleen and my medical teams noticed my behavior changed. I was impatient with people, causing Paul R to ask if I was depressed. I said I was not depressed, just not feeling myself.

My friend and Dana clinical trial nurse, Debby D, suggested it could be a thyroid problem. Tests confirmed her judgment, again showing the importance of each team member.

In 2019, I experienced another possible side effect of long-time cancer or treatments which lowered my immune system. I had 2 cases of pneumonia and each was difficult. One lung had fluid that required removal, and more days in the hospital. Marcos and Paul R believe my risk of another virus, like pneumonia, is higher than my risk for my cancers' returning. I do everything I can to avoid another uncomfortable pneumonia episode or worse.

Due to the pneumonia, GVHD or something else, my legs swelled significantly which made walking difficult. I could not ride my bike for the POHR. Something caused a hip or muscle injury near one hip, making it impossible to walk. I was in a wheelchair for a few weeks before slowly walking with crutches and then a cane for about a month. My medical team advised that in time my mobility would return, and they were right.

These 2019 experiences give me heightened respect for avoiding another virus. Pneumonia in my situation is a significant and serious risk. I began taking IVIG treatments to strengthen my immune system, as other myeloma patients also do.

Whether or not caused by cancer or my treatments, I had another adverse effect. I experienced difficulty controlling anger. It surfaced over an insignificant situation when I overreacted and caused my family and me unneeded pain. It was not who I was, and help was needed. I asked Bob K and followed his advice and consulted with a veteran UH professional counselor. This was a difficult, but necessary, decision.

Counseling sessions helped me understand what causes my anger, and more importantly, practical actions I continue drawing upon to better manage myself. I am grateful my family relationships were restored.

Was it Worth it ?

Hell yes, it was well worth the treatments, hospitalization, and stress on both of us and our families. Being with my family enabled me to be part of many great memories I thought I would never have.

Being with Kathleen for many more years after I was diagnosed, supporting one another, and enjoying being together, whether family vacations, seeing parts of the country and the world, family birthdays, anniversaries, golfing on Sunday afternoons, surprising her on her 70th birthday with our expanded families and closest friends, celebrating our 50th wedding anniversary, being with her when she received the ACS's highest volunteer award, or just relaxing together.

Being with our sons at their weddings, seeing grandchildren arrive, being with Jillian when she played sports in the backyard, being with Dayton and Wade when they caught their first fish, being surprised when Jim took me to Scotland for my 60th birthday, watching Bob's basketball team win the state championship, and being with our sons at Cleveland Indians World Series games.

Being with my sisters and their children, being with Becki and Dan when their daughter Amy hosted their 50th wedding anniversary, being with Denyse and Charlie for my surprise 70th birthday, which their daughter, Mandy, hosted and I was given a compilation of family pictures which Stacey, Emilee and others made happen.

Being with my father and father-in-law while they were still with us, saltwater fishing trips with Kathleen's father, and earlier Canadian fishing trips with my dad, and more recently with my good friend, Roy Burnett.

Golfing with my family for twenty years in the Janell B. Izzo annual golf outing, which her husband, Charlie, founded and led.

Sharing Our Story

Sharing our survival story became part of our lives. It started in 1993 when Bob K invited me to say a few words at an ACS Hope Lodge fundraising event. Bob explained to the group of women how cancer research enabled my first transplant, and why more funding is needed to give more patients access to major cancer centers who performed transplants. As a recent stem cell transplant patient, I stepped up to the podium and shared highlights of our first year living with cancer.

I recall being amazed with what happened when I ended. Several women walked up towards me before I could leave the podium. I thought my comments must have meant a lot to them. But when they got to the podium, they turned and headed for Kathleen who was sitting in the front row. They were hugging her and getting emotional, providing comfort for all she went through as my care giver. This event also helped start Kathleen's ACS volunteer career, first with our Hope Lodge, and eventually to the ACS

Board of Directors in Atlanta, and earn virtually every ACS volunteer leadership award.

A couple years later, a UH orthopedic doctor's wife was diagnosed with myeloma, and he asked us to share our experiences. He and his wife came to our house, and we ended the conversation over two hours later. When they left, we looked at each other and we both had the same reaction. We had hoped that sharing our story may help the other couple, but we did not expect it also would help us.

Paul R asked me to do an interview with Newsweek magazine after my life-saving response to the Velcade clinical trial. My goal in doing the interview was to provide some hope to other myeloma patients and their families. The son of a woman newly-diagnosed with myeloma contacted me after the article, and we became friends with his mother and father and shared information for years. Another woman saw the article and thanked me before we shared our story at a fundraiser. She said her young daughter was recently diagnosed with myeloma, and our story gave her needed hope.

Many years ago, at a UH volunteer gathering, the cancer center leader Dr. Jim Willson advised me to make use of the platform he believed we have. We have tried to do this, especially with the value of clinical trials.

We have shared our story over 250 times in over 35 states, National Academy of Sciences in Washington, DC., Canada, Japan, and Spain. Almost all involved trips to cancer groups; some were podcasts for myeloma and other foundations and others were webinars (or webcasts). And some were videos posted to their sites or YouTube.

At one support group in Rochester, MN we were honored that Dr. Robert Kyle, a legend in multiple myeloma, who wrote the book on myeloma years ago, attended to hear our story. We had met Bob before and exchanged information with him. The support group leader indicated it was the first time he attended.

On the same trip, we took time to visit one of Kathleen's high school friends, Susan, who had sung in our wedding.

More recently, we avoid travel by sharing our story virtually. I cover patient and Kathleen covers caregiver experiences. We do not offer medical advice, just our experiences.

In 2004, my EY leader suggested we could reach more people worldwide by working with the firm's webcast team and a myeloma foundation and do a webcast. He assured me the firm supported this use of our resources. After selecting three other myeloma patients who were in a speaking program we were in, I served as moderator and panelist and Kathleen was behind the scenes, selecting the questions from listeners. The first question was from our son, Jim, who recently pointed out this webcast likely was the first by myeloma patients. The webcast was posted to the firm's site and viewed by several hundred around the world.

Luck

Some hear our story and tell me, "Jim, you are just lucky."

I agree with them, I am a very lucky person. Having my parents, Jim and Delores Bond, raise me was very lucky. They worked tirelessly to give all four of their children a better life. They demonstrated the unequalled value of hard work and not giving up despite setbacks. Most of all they gave us their love. I miss them.

I am very lucky to have three wonderful sisters, and grateful to Becki for donating her stem cells and for Denyse for her unwavering support and for Janell's love while she was with us. Their husbands, Dan and Charlie, are two of my best friends, as is Janell's surviving spouse, Charlie. I am also lucky they each have children that support us.

I am lucky to have had the support of Kathleen's parents, Bob and Mae, and her siblings, Robert, Don, and Mary Ann, and John.

My mother's parents passed away when I was young, but I was very lucky to have my grandfather, Dayton R Bond, spend lots of time giving me a better appreciation of the outdoors and the value of compromise without adversity.

I am lucky to have spent over 50 years married to Kathleen, a remarkable person. And we have been blessed to have Jim and Emilee, Bob and Stacey, and grandchildren, Dayton, Wade and Jillian

I also believe the following about our luck in surviving two cancers. A now departed golf instructor in Texas would explain luck to his collegiate golfers, essentially in these terms:

When you are facing a very long putt across an undulating green, you *are* lucky if you sink the putt in one stroke. But the key is to hit the ball hard enough to get it to the hole, and thereby *give luck a chance to happen*.

We try to do all we can to give luck a chance to happen. By taking time to read our story, and others, you may be giving yourself a better chance for luck to happen.

Kathleen would end by adding, "And watch out for those *pink Buicks.*"

Acronyms for Patients and Caregivers

I developed acronyms that summarize much of our approach to cancer: for patients, RESPECT ALL, and for caregivers SLEEP LATER which stand for:

Read, or research, myeloma from credible sources
Exercise daily, a little or a lot; "sit, stand, walk;"" Stay on your feet not your seat"
Second opinions when appropriate
Partner with your medical team
Each case is unique
Comply with agreed instructions & dosage
Trials (clinical trials) when appropriate

Always ask your medical team if you need help
Long-term plans are important
Luck can happen, give it a chance

For caregivers:

Stories can help, like our 007 story
Let go emotionally when needed

Eight PM Rule - no cancer talk after 8 p.m.

Exercise and stay healthy

Pink Buick story gives perspective

Look ahead, looking back not helpful

Always do the necessary, then the possible, may do impossible

Take care of yourself first

Exercise can be therapeutic

Rapidly things can change, never give up

Acknowledgements and Thanks to:

My wife, Kathleen, for her insights and help with this book, and to our daughter-in-law, Stacey Bond, who graciously offered to review and offer suggestions along with her husband, Bob.

Our sons, James E and Robert D Bond, and their wives, Emilee and Stacey and children, Dayton, Wade and Jillian for their unwavering support and encouragement.

My sister, Becki Kramer her husband Dan Kramer, a best friend, and their children, Matt, Steve, and Amy for their unwavering support. Becki's matching stem cells saved my life, as did her platelets years later.

My sister Denyse Patterson and her husband Charlie, a best friend, and their son Chuck and daughter Mandy Highland and her children, Jack, and Claire. Mandy hosted my 70th birthday party. Their unwavering support and encouragement inspired me.

My brother-in-law and good friend, Charlie Izzo, my departed sister, Janell's husband. Charlie's 20 year memorial golf tournament is one example of his generous support in the fight against cancer.

Kathleen's parents, Robert E and Mae Mercer and Kathleen's brothers, Robert G, Don, John and sister, Mary Ann John and their children. Kathleen's father and brother Don enabled special transportation to get us to Dana Farber for the Velcade clinical trial. Her brother John looked after our home when we were in Boston for 9 months during the same trial. Her sister Mary Ann solved my technical issues while doing a recorded interview.

My friends and authors, Doug Geib and Paul Lepp, for their book insights.

Our good friends: Sally and Dan O'Brien, Myia and Jack Sterling, Theresa Daher Roy Burnett, Dennis Hoffer and Rick Barnhart for their support.

The American Cancer Society and its CEO Gary Reedy, former CEO John Seffrin, PhD. and executive staff, Our Pan Ohio Hope Ride leaders Sarah Morris and Stacy McGrath, Paul Purdy, ACS Endurance Events Manager, ACS Ohio staff, and many volunteers and riders. The ACS arranged for us to tell our story in many cities, at the National Academy of Sciences in Washington, DC, and the ACS has made several videos of our story.

My Ernst & Young (EY) good friends, including Marilyn Willis, Jim Breitenbach, Walt Avdey, Mike Beihl, Bob Callan, Chuck Hauser, Jim Mach, Jim Boland, Ron Hill, Dennis Jancsy, Darrell Schubert, Sven Lang, Jack Poldruhi, Denise Weber, Scott Merk, Randy Anstine, Sue Flis, and Arthur Spector, who visited my transplant room after work on a Friday to solve technical issues with my EY laptop. It meant a lot.

My good client friends, the late Jerry Weinberger, John Brinzo, Bob Leroux, Dave Costa, Clark Waite, Bill Ladika, Craig and Brian Koenig, Bob Lovejoy, Ray Miller, John Lupo, Ren Carlisle, Vince Coneglio, and Jack Horner.

Our friends at Takeda Oncology (and its predecessor Millennium Pharmaceutical): Shawn Goodman, Julian Adams, Dixie Esseltine, David Schenkein, Ronny Mosston, Janice Berman, Kathy Gram, Sabina McCafferty, Phil Soro, Fatima Scipione and Brent

Evans. Takeda helped enable us to share our story in 33 states and Japan.

International Myeloma Foundation and support group leaders, Cynthia Ralston and Stephanie McCrae, and founder, Susie Duric (Novis). The IMF enabled us to visit many US support groups and virtually share our story with 10 more IMF support groups, including a webinar for Canada IMF. The IMF helped enable us to say a few words in Spain to help honor Paul Richardson for receiving the prestigious Robert A. Kyle Lifetime Achievement Award.

Leukemia, Lymphoma, (and myeloma) Society and its leader, Meg Boyko. The LLS posted an interview on its website.

National Bone Marrow Transplant and its leader, Peggy Burkhard. The NBMT interviewed us and posted it on its site. And its affiliated Be the Match site for donors to register.

Myeloma Crowd and its founder, Jenny Ahlstrom, who interviewed us and posted these on its site.

Patient Power and its founder, Andrew Schorr who interviewed us and posted these on its site.

The Multiple Myeloma Research Foundation (MMRF) for use of its mailing list which our EY team used to broadcast the groundbreaking myeloma patient webcast seen live or recorded by several hundreds of patients worldwide. EY's Joan Dollard-Spooner led our team. I selected three patient panelists (Bruce H, Angie M, and Torrance C.), wrote a script, and served as a panelist. EY generously funded the webcast. Kathleen screened live questions.

Myeloma patients and friends who traded ongoing experiences with me: Dave S, Ernie W, Joyce S, Bob S, Tony P, Pat K, Cindy C. and Chris S. Hundreds of patients around the world who contacted me and exchanged survival experiences.

Doctors and Nurses of University Hospitals of Cleveland and its Seidman Cancer Center:

Drs. Bob Kellermeyer, Marcos deLima, and their transplant team. And, Drs. Kevin Geraci, William Petersilge and Ivan Cakulev.

Nurses Ann Kolenik, Rose Miller, Tina Shin, Lee Shetina, Linda Baer, Nina Dambrosio, and Leslie Craig

University Hospitals interviewed us multiple times and posted these on its site.

Dana Farber Cancer Institute: Drs. Paul Richardson, Rob Schlossman, Ken Anderson, and Dan DeAngelo

Nurses Debbie Doss, Mary McKenny and Kathy Colson

Dana Farber invited us to share our story many times at its annual myeloma symposium events, and posted these on its site. Thanks to Jack Sparacino and Katie Kupferberg

Mayo Clinic: the late Dr. Philip Greipp and retired Dr. Robert Kyle, the 'Father of Myeloma 'to many of us

Massachusetts General Hospital: Dr. Tom Spitzer

BostonSight: Dr. Allan Kwok and technician Heidi Wolfe

Cleveland Clinic Cancer Center—Diagnosing Doctor Dr. Alan Lichten

Praise for Jim and Kathleen Bond

"James Bond's 2002 Velcade clinical trial saved his life. Being my most compliant patient also played a vital role in his success."
Robert W. Kellermeyer, MD. University Hospitals of Cleveland Seidman Cancer Center

"I have learned so much from Jim and Kathleen. I have witnessed the wisdom of Jim's persistence, belief and amazing courage. I have shared Kathleen's important advocacy and coping tips with many patients."
Deborah Doss, RN. OCN

"I remember Jim's appointment with us before heading to Boston, the weather was mild but he arrived in a winter coat. Jim was quite ill and I thought I probably would not see him again. But with his incredible will to live, he made it to Boston and entered a cutting-edge clinical trial that resulted in Velcade.

I recall he was Patient 007. Due to brave patients like Jim enrolling in clinical trials Velcade became the first new medication for myeloma. We no longer had to start with toxic chemotherapy, and this led to better initial response rates."
Rose Miller, RN.

"I began caring for Jim 29 years ago at his diagnosis and continued for many years. Jim and Kathleen's story is one of amazing advocacy, perseverance, love and strength. The hope and inspiration they bring to others is extraordinary. They have both influenced patient cancer care throughout the country."
Ann Kolenic, PhD, DNP, APRN, AOCNS

"For 10 years I have been honored to know Jim and Kathleen Bond, first as a patient/caregiver team and then as patient advocates. Their commitment to supporting, teaching, and fundraising for patients and families affected by cancer is amazing. The work they have done through the American Cancer Society is inspiring."
Nina Dambrosio, RN, CNP

"Jim is a mental force to be reckoned with. We met in 2006 when Kathleen and I were putting together the initial American Cancer Society Pan Ohio Hope Ride

for 2007. Jim was one of our novices, never riders who bought a bike, trained and despite being frail from cancer treatments he cycled 328 miles in 4 days, including a 100-mile day. 'Superman' Jim cycles 7 - 9 mph, taking 12+ hours some days. Day 3, Arriving at Antioch College sweat pouring into his eyes, he did not see his fellow riders waiting for him and kept pedaling, personifying his character and willpower. I cherish the times we have ridden together. I proudly call Jim and Kathleen my friends who have truly enriched my life."
Dennis Hoffer, Rider #1, POHR Co-Founder

CPSIA information can be obtained
at www.ICGtesting.com
Printed in the USA
BVHW070850231121
622335BV00005B/135